£2.00

CW00661360

ACUPUNCTURE HANDBOOK

ACUPUNCTURE
HANDBOOK

by

Denis Lawson-Wood

and

Joyce Lawson-Wood

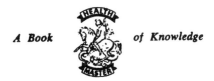

A Book   *of Knowledge*

HEALTH SCIENCE PRESS
Denington Estate, Wellingborough
Northamptonshire

First published 1964
Second revised Edition, March 1973

ISBN 0 85032 105 0

Printed in Great Britain by
Straker Brothers Ltd., Whitstable

CONTENTS

PREFACE

The typescript of this present work was completed and in the publisher's hands before the end of 1959. Owing to unavoidable delays of one sort and another, over which neither we nor the publishers had any control, it was not found possible to publish this work until 1964. In the intervening years two things have happened of great importance to those interested in Chinese Acupuncture, especially to those intending to study with a view to practise.

(i)   The Research Society for Naturopathy has been active in investigating the therapeutic potentialities of Chinese Acupuncture, testing instrumental detection of the Meridians and Points, and organizing a Study Course for practitioners. Electronic instruments are now available to practitioners, and it is now possible to confirm scientifically the reality of the Meridians and Points by meter readings and the 'magic eye'. We have our own instrument, with which we are experimenting, made specially for us according to a circuit designed by Kenneth Morgan. With this instrument, in lieu of meter readings and the 'magic eye', detection is by means of variations in intensity of sound. As with some of the other instruments, ours can also be used for treatment.

(ii)   Other publications in English are now available, the most important of these being Dr. Lavier's work on Chinese Acupuncture (published by the Health Science Press). At the present day Dr. Lavier must undoubtedly be considered as *the* leading authority in Europe on the Traditional Chinese Acupuncture. His intimate knowledge of the Chinese Language has enabled him to go direct to source for information and facts; it is therefore no longer necessary to rely on translations coloured by translators' prejudices and/or misconceptions.

We do earnestly ask of our readers that they will not forget the date of the writing of this our present work when evaluating the matter therein.

PREFACE TO SECOND EDITION

We may perhaps never learn how acupuncture points were first so accurately located at least four thousand five hundred years ago: and, from some points of view, it is of relatively little importance now that we not only have the tradition, but also successful verification of traditional placing of points and paths linking them has begun. Modern scientific research has already produced factual evidence of such a nature that not even the most sceptical is justified in dismissing acupuncture as fanciful or superstitious nonsense. It is even becoming quite respectable to be interested in acupuncture. The wide publicity being given, through television, to its use as an anaesthetic brings to my mind the following passage from Dr. Ilza Veith's introduction to the Nei Ching:

'... It was not entirely the superiority of Chinese internal medicine that made surgery unnecessary, but the Confucian tenets of the sacredness of the body, which counteracted any tendency toward the development of anatomical studies and the practice of surgery. Nevertheless, Chinese medical history records two eminent surgeons, Pien Ch'iao and Hua T'o. Pien Ch'iao practised in the second century B.C., and legend ascribes to him such skilful use of anaesthesia that he was able to operate painlessly and even to exchange successfully the hearts of two patients. Hua T'o, whose writings on surgery and anaesthesia became known around 190 A.D., is definitely established as an historical personality, famous for his excellent operative technique.'

Although I had learned the traditional placing of points; needle, moxa and massage techniques; used this knowledge in practice over the years without really understanding 'what worked, how or why, but nevertheless did', it was not until the end of 1965 that answers to the What? How? Why? began to reach me from behind the Iron Curtain.

I managed to obtain copies of a Report delivered by Professor Kim Bong Han at a scientific symposium in

Pyongyang November 30th 1963; and two papers read by him at the first scientific symposium of the Korean Society of Kyungrak held in Pyongyang on April 15th 1965. (Published by the Medical Science Press, Pyongyang, Korea).

In Chinese Medicine Tradition there are about eight hundred known acupuncture points on the human body: at these points action may be taken by needle, moxa, massage, etc., to treat particular disease conditions. Some points are forbidden to the needle as, for example, a point on the arm known as 'Blue Death'; a needle here can stop heart action. Some points are forbidden to moxa as, for example, certain points on the face near the eyes. A few points are forbidden to both needle and moxa, e.g., a point on the median posterior line between D.10 and D.11.

In spite of well over one hundred years of Western Medicine propaganda, the setting up of Western Medicine Hospitals and so on, Western and Eastern medicine remained far apart. Sad to say, adherents of Western Schools tended always to adopt a somewhat supercilious superiority attitude towards the native practitioners. Fortunately a change is now taking place as a result of the sensible and courageous step taken by the appropriate authorities of the Democratic Peoples' Republic of Korea in setting up a research team to enquire into acupuncture.

The research team, led by Professor Kim Bong Han, was provided with adequate funds, all requisite modern scientific equipment and, above all, given official encouragement throughout long years of hard work, difficulties and frustrations.

The outcome has been most rewarding: the team having made discoveries of such importance to biology and medical science that more than one of the generally accepted theories and prevailing notions will have to be re-assessed.

The two major accomplishments of the Bong Han team are:

(1) Demonstrating the existence of the independent functional-morphological system known traditionally in Korean as the Kyungrak system. It is now experimentally verified and established that at the traditional acupuncture points (known in Korean medicine as the Kyunghyul positions) there exists an hitherto unknown and unsuspected structure now named a Bonghan Corpuscle; and, linking the

corpuscles, there is a system of ducts following exactly the traditional pathways or meridians through which a fluid circulates.

(2) Experimental results of research into the function and role of the system of corpuscles and ducts; and into the composition of Bonghan fluid make it imperative that the current cell theory (i.e. that the cell is the unitary morphological and functional unit of the organism, and that cells are formed only from cells through division, etc.) be re-examined with a view to re-formulation.

First about the Bonghan corpuscles and ducts: Bonghan corpuscles are not only to be found in the dermis at the Kyunghyul positions (acupuncture points) but they are to be found widely distributed in the profunda of the organism. There are some differences between the superficial and the profound corpuscles, as for example, the superficial corpuscle consists of an outer layer of smooth muscle and an inner substance made up of various cells, whereas the deep corpuscle has no outer muscle layer. Histo-chemical and biochemical studies show that the corpuscle inner substance has an abundance of desoxyribonucleic acid (DNA). It can scarcely be too often emphasized that the corpuscle structure is completely different from any other structure hitherto known; and to some extent so also are the ducts linking the corpuscles. The ducts are made up of bundles of ductules consisting of endothelial cells of single layer forming a very soft thin wall.

Ducts linking corpuscles are either intra- or extravascular. That is to say ducts run inside blood or lymphatic vessels or they do not: here we note two important features: (i) Wherever there is a blood or lymphatic vessel there is an internal Bonghan duct, and (ii) the direction of flow of the fluid in the duct is usually the same as the blood flow but not always.

As regards the extra vascular ducts, these are to be found (a) distributed on the surface of organs independently of blood and lymphatic vessels or nerves: (b) running along the outer surface of the walls of blood and lymphatic vessels or along nerves; and (c) distributed in the Central and in the Peripheral Nervous System, running inside the central canal of the spinal cord and the cerebral ventricles.

It will be realized from the foregoing that the ducts form

a vast network distributed all over the body, its organs, glands, muscles, ramifying into connective tissues, etc. But the Bonghan duct system has no such centre as the heart; neither are the ducts linked to form a single route; but the Bonghan fluid has many routes EACH LINKED with a DIFFERENT Organ, exactly coinciding with tradition. Nevertheless all the systems of Kyungrak are interlinked to form ONE INTEGRATED System.

Traditionally the superficial ducts and corpuscles form Twelve bi-lateral and two median circuits: each of the twelve being associated with and named after an inner organ.

The 1963 paper and the first 1965 paper should be studied in order to appreciate the general structure of the Bonghan ducts and corpuscles: the various systems and their roles: Biochemical composition of the Bonghan fluid (e.g. Nitrogen, Sugar, Lipid, Hyaluronic acid, and free amino acid content; and the base composition of DNA and nucleotide composition of RNA): and the Bioelectrical features and effect of stimuli to ducts and corpuscles.

We now turn our attention to the second major accomplishment of the Bong Han team: The Theory of Sanal. This is the subject of the second paper read by the professor in 1965: the introduction to this is now quoted in full.

'In the course of studying the physiological functions of the Kyungrak system, a new anatomico-histological system in the organism, we have come to realize the new important facts which underlie all the phenomena of life. We have ascertained that unique granules (they are named "Bonghan Sanal" after the discoverer) circulate in the Kyungrak system and they grow into cells, and that the cells of organs and tissues turn into the Bonghan Sanal, while moving through the Kyungrak system.

This process is repeated in a continuous cycle. (This cyclic process is called "Bonghan Sanal-cell cycle").

Through the research into the continuous process of the Bonghan Sanal-cell cycle, we have come to form the following new views on the self-renovation of the organism.

1. **All the Morphological Constituent Parts of the Organism Are Incessantly Renewed.**

2. **The Self-renovation of the Organism Takes the Form of Bonghan Sanal-cell Cycle.**

3. The Self-renovation of the Organism is Performed by the Kyungrak System.

We name these views "Theory of Sanal". A series of researches have been performed to prove the validity of these views. Results obtained are presented here.

The Theory of Sanal, of course, requires the re-examination of the cell theory and other cardinal problems of biology.'

One member of a group of doctors to whom I was lecturing commented with a shrug of his shoulders and an undisguised sneer: 'Until all that theory has been properly verified it is worth no more than science fiction or a huge hoax.' But that was five years ago.

Today the accumulated publicity, given in particular to the anaesthetic use of acupuncture points, has raised this Far-Oriental Tradition well above fanciful superstition. We are now, however, excused from exercising reasonable caution before acceptance of new claims and new theories. It seems to me that NOW is the time for acupuncture, Kyungrak, and the Theory of Sanal, to be thoroughly investigated by unprejudiced researchers adequately equipped. The field is wide enough to keep many teams busy for several decades. The term 'unprejudiced' here means more than 'impartial', it is intended to include the notion 'ability and willingness to think on unaccustomed levels'.

One hundred and fifty years ago Hahnemann was continually faced with the difficulty of persuading students (and colleagues) to *think* in terms of *homoeopathic* remedies and dosage and NOT in terms of minute doses of *allopathic* remedies. Items in one system cannot be properly assessed in terms of a different system. (One does not measure milk by the yard). Homoeopathy is mentioned here because, in our view, there may eventually be found a strong link with acupuncture. It would be wise, however, in their early studies of Chinese acupuncture to think as simply and whole-heartedly as possible the 'Chinese way'.

As an example of the folly of mixing methods that I actually witnessed: A practitioner injecting a minute dose of an aperient at the acupuncture 'constipation point'! As this point is on the first finger it can readily be appreciated that the allopathic aperient had no effect..The use of that kind of needle at this point was, from the chinese acupuncture viewpoint, quite wrong. In one case of measles, child age 12, very high temperature and at least three days constipated, I massaged that point on the finger with a 'bone needle' for ten seconds only. Within fifteen minutes temperature had dropped one degree, and within twenty minutes there was a substantial bowel movement.

The differences between Eastern and Western medicine are so great that it should be obvious that 'thinking-patterns' must also be very different.

Where the western doctor feels *the* pulse the eastern doctor recognizes *twelve* pulses.

The Far-oriental doctor recognizes the blood-circulation network as an organ: he also recognizes a temperature regulation organ which he calls the 'Three Burning Spaces'. Ideally, as a superior doctor, his interest is predominantly prophyllactic: and it is only the 'inferior doctor' who concerns himself with palliatives and surgery: whereas in the West the interests are reversed.

The Yellow Emperor's Classic of Internal Medicine looks with horror upon a civilization which feeds its young with white sugar until the teeth rot and then puts fluoride into the nation's drinking water to enable the folly to continue.

To new researchers we say that it looks as if the field opened up by Kim Bong Han offers highly rewarding possibilities, especially as regards controlling proliferation of tumour cells. Many conditions now little understood and considered incurable may become clear, and treatments discovered.

Well! There is the challenge!

INTRODUCTION

This present work is intended to serve the dual purpose, Study and Reference.

First and foremost we aim to put before the English speaking people a simple and reasonably comprehensive amount of information on the subject of Acupuncture, sufficient to enable anyone interested in this ancient system of healing from the Far East to practise the art; or at the least to make a good beginning. With this in mind we have arranged the material in such a way as to make study simple and progressive. Enough primary notions of Yang-Yin Science are given in the early pages for a thoughtful reader thoroughly to grasp the general principles upon which the science is based. Then, in logical order, we present some factors to be taken into consideration in assessment of the requirements in any particular case (danger signals, pulses, etc.).

The points for treatment are arranged in groups; each group is, where convenient, sub-divided into sections so that by studying and memorising but one sub-division at a time (if one wishes to commit the points to memory) and by alloting one week for each such sub-division the principal points can be learned in about six months: though, undoubtedly, there will be many who will find that they can proceed more rapidly.

• We then follow on with an outline of treatment methods and repertory. The repertory is intended only as a guide and should not be looked upon as complete. Each individual practitioner will develop his own personal technique as he progresses in skill and artistry, and discover couplings and combinations of points.

Secondly this book is designed for rapid reference. The grouping of points, sub-divisions of groups, and so on, should make it a simple matter to turn up information required.

Wherever we have come across differences of opinion among authoritative writers on acupuncture regarding the positioning of points we have elected, as in our previous work*, to follow the numbering, positioning, and nomenclature of Doctor Roger de la Fuÿe: ** this we have done, not necessarily because of one hundred

* Chinese System of Healing, Health Science Press, 1959.
**Traiteć d'Acupuncture (le François, 1956)

per cent agreement with him, but because we feel that as Dr. de la Fuÿe has had so many years study of the subject coupled with years and years of *clinical experience,* during which he has verified points and their homœopathic remedy correspondences, his conclusions should be treated with the greatest respect and may safely be followed until one is in a position, after comparable work, to confirm, modify, or replace them.

Laborious comparing of ancient and modern texts might well help one to arrive at one or another *traditional* placing and nature of a point; but the verdict of tradition is not necessarily the soundest. We do not consider that one need feel disturbed by the fact that authorities sometimes disagree, for, in our view, the mere fact of disagreement appears relatively insignificant by comparison with the *reasons* for any such disagreement. When the *reasons* have been understood it will frequently be found that what appeared to be a disagreement (even a contradiction) turns out not to be: for one finds that other factors, not previously taken into account, put a different complexion on the matter. Slavish following of any one tradition, however time-honoured, may just as easily be a slavish perpetuating of one or more errors as of one or more empirically verifiable facts. Understanding of principles is to be arrived at through contemplation and ordered thinking — not through psittacotic learning.

The matter of making adequate acknowledgements of sources of information presented something of a problem to us; we realized that what might be looked upon as adequate by some would be considered inadequate by others. When one's *reading* life has extended over forty years or more it seems a hopeless task to try and remember all the books one has read on any subject, or exactly where particular items of information were acquired. As an example we have studied at least three English translations of the Tao Teh King; two of them so long ago that we cannot recall the names of translators or publishers, nor even from which library or person we borrowed them. Though we owe much to those works we cannot mention them by name, and we have to content ourselves by referring to the translation now on our bookshelves*.

From our teens and twenties to the present day we have read several hundred books on Eastern Philosophies, Religions, and Sciences, some cursorily, some meticulously: to all we owe something. To us it appears irrelevant to name them all (even could we remember them all); even more irrelevant does it appear to us to consider the vast mass of reading matter dating back to our first ABC and Childhood Reading Primer: nevertheless we owe something to each and every one, and, of course, to all we have heard in the course of talks, lectures, or private oral tuition. Some works seem to come into the category of 'obviously relevant', as for example the works of Doctors Roger de la Fuÿe, Erich W. Stiefvater, Nyoiti Saku-razawa, Nakayama, and so on, as well as references to ancient texts; acknowledgement appears in the form of Footnotes.

* The Way and Its Power, A Study of the Tao Tê Ching and Its Place in Chinese Thought, by Arthur Waley, George Allen and Unwin Ltd., 1934.

In between the obviously relevant and irrelevant are those which one finds difficult to decide whether to include or not. No two people will have exactly the same ideas as to where the relevant begins or ends. In order to ensure that at least implicit acknowledgement is made to everyone to whom it should be made we offer this Dedication:—

TO OUR TWO SONS,

JULIAN and ADRIAN,

AND ALL GENERATIONS AS YET

UNBORN

AS A TOKEN OF

DEEP GRATITUDE FOR OUR INHERITANCE:

THE FRUITS

OF THE EFFORTS, TOIL AND DARING

OF ALL

PAST GENERATIONS

FROM THE FIRST MAN—ADAM

THEORY AND PRACTICE

I

During the last fifty years Acupuncture has become widely known and practised on the Continent, and is looked upon as "orthodox and respectable". To this present day, however, there is still no adequate nor comprehensive western scientific theory (as far as we are aware) to explain why Acupuncture works; there is thus a vast field open to research workers who are able to orient their thinking in line with the most up-to-date (1960) scientific method, and who are ready to delve into new theories as and when they come along.

In order to grasp the philosophic notions and scientific theory upon which Acupuncture is based one does not need to study the Chinese language, nor even to read translations of Chinese philosophic writings of antiquity. It is possible, we feel, to acquire and cultivate the necessary habitual orientation by the careful study of one or more of the excellent and simple text books published in recent years on modern thinking method, for these prepare the mind by cultivating flexibility in thinking*, after which one should go on

* Explorations in Awareness, J. Samuel Bois, Harper 1957
Language Habits in Human Affairs, Irving J. Lee, Harper 1941
Your Most Enchanted Listener, Wendell Johnson, Harper 1957

to the *thorough* study of Korzybski's works* and Dr. Swanson's

* Science & Sanity by Alfred Korzybski, 3rd ed 1948, published by the Institute of General Semantics, Lakeville, Connecticut, USA., and Time-Binding The General Theory, two papers by Korzybski (1924 & 1926) in one volume 1954.

Lectures on Electro-colloidal Structures**, which bring up-to-date

**General Semantics Monograph IV by M. Swanson, 1959, published by the Institute of General Semantics.

the chapters on non-elementalistic structures in Korzybski's Science & Sanity. For those who read French we strongly recommend Sakurazawa's Principe Unique***.

***Principe Unique de la Philosophie et de la Science d'Extrême-Orient, Nyoiti Sakurazawa, (J. Vrin, Paris, 1958).

The most advanced methods of current scientific thinking seem to indicate a trend closely allied to the formulations of FOU-HI* (circa 2950 BC), and to those of HERACLITUS the Ionian philosopher (540-475 BC).

* Sakurawa, op.cit.

Heraclitus observed the fundamental fact that everywhere in nature everything changes incessantly; everything both IS and IS NOT at one and the same time: Harmony and Unity consist in diversity and multiplicity. The sole actuality is an eternal flux and change: all phenomena are in a state of continuous transition from non-existence to existence and from existence to non-existence. He talks of *two forces* working in all things: a force that moves them on the upward path to "fire", and an opposite force that moves them on the downward path to "earth". All existence, he declares, whatever its state or form, is the result of dynamic balancing of these opposing forces: and nature, as a whole, represents an eternal oscillation between them.

Western Culture has waited until this XXth Century AD for the development of that principle of relativity arrived at by Heraclitus 2500 years before Einstein—a principle which was known in the Far-East to FOU-HI yet another 2500 years *before* Heraclitus.

FOU-HI was a tireless observer of nature who arrived at the conclusion that the fundamental phenomenon was *Rythmic Change*. He observed that everything evolves; that is to say, is in a state of continuous change; all things and happenings are linked, dependant and interdependant; all existence is a manifestation of the interplay of *two forces,* YANG and YIN.

YANG represents the force of FULNESS: it is compressive, cohesive, constrictive, centripetal, attracting, implosive, solidifying, crystallizing, etc.

2

YIN represents the negative force which functions as the dilating, repelling, centrifugal, expansive, explosive, liquifying, dispersing polarity.

These two forces, YANG and YIN, represent the two poles of the Unitary Force; and the Space-Time world happens as a result of polarization of the Unitary Force and the perpetual interplay of these two polarities weaving and inter-weaving in complexities of infinitely diverse patternings.

    * Speaking at the Attingham Park Conference, 1959, Sir George Trevelyan, Warden of Attingham Park, said: "The whole of life turns on polarities, on antagonistic pulls. It is as if an elastic were stretched out. You can't keep the tension unless you keep the pull. The very life of the elastic turns on the antagonism. The whole working of the human organism, which is near the whole of nature, turns on the sustaining of the antagonistic pulls. . . . The world of thought is a great whole. Moving forwards, we are part of it . . . and every one of us according to the power of our perception, the background of our experience, has obviously something to contribute, the best of our own intergrity and vision. . . . The evolutionary concept can and should be applied to our thinking, to our consciousness, which is all part of a great evolving pattern. Apparent conflicts gain their meaning, not their resolution, by being recognized as complementary to each other in this state of tension and antagonism which is life." Extracts from the article by Helen Murray in Mother Earth, October 1959 (The quarterly publication of the Soil Association).

The Origin of all that exists is Pure Abstract Unitary Principle Static; existence is polarization without beginning and without end, hence "creation" is continuous (dynamic embodiment)*.

    * compare with a "modern re-discovery" of these principles as set forth by C. W. Davson, M.I.Mech.E., M.Inst.Pet., in The Physics of the Primary State of Matter, (Elverton Books) 1955.

Nothing is neutral. Nothing is *wholly* YANG nor wholly YIN, but only relatively so. Every Being, Thing, or Circumstance represents YANG-YIN interplay. This is illustrated in the well known symbol: —

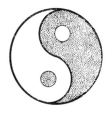

It should be carefully noted that the large shaded area contains a small circle unshaded; and the large unshaded area contains a small shaded circle. Unless these two small areas within the large are depicted *the symbol is incomplete*: for these serve as symbolic representations of the fact that nothing is *wholly* either Yang or Yin: however small the proportion of Yang within Yin or Yin within Yang some *there must be*. This we can illustrate by referring to the recognition, by both Eastern and Western scientists, of the need for the co-existence in all forms of plant, animal, and human life of certain *trace-elements without which a plant, etc., dies*. Two essential trace elements are Potassium (K.) representative of YIN and Sodium (Na.) representative of YANG.

In health the vital bi-polar (*Yang-Yin*) force called TSRI flows smoothly, freely throughout the organism in dynamic equilibrium. *All* sickness, slight or serious, is but a manifestation of a *disturbed* YANG-YIN equilibrium; all healing art, therefore, is directed towards the restoration of normal YANG-YIN balance. Here, and throughout this book, we use the term *normal* to mean standard or "what it *should* be"; *by normal we do not mean average.*

To the Far-Eastern healing practitioner the art lies not in the treatment of diseases once they have become manifested externally (or overtly) in more or less distressing symptoms, but in *foreseeing* the probable long-term consequences of present YANG-YIN imbalance *if left untreated*. The Chinese practitioner anticipates and treats a disease before it happens; thus preventing it from ever happening. This does not mean to say, of course, that he is any less able than his Western colleague to deal with diseases, sicknesses, and derangements that do become manifested; for, obviously, there is always the possibility of unforeseen emergencies such as accident, epidemic, and so on.

Acupuncture-point therapy is based on the hypothesis that TSRI, the vital bi-polar (Yang-Yin) force circulates rhythmically throughout the organism and permeates every cell and tissue in the body. The complete circuit is made every twenty-four hours*. The main flow is in certain traditionally established paths *traceable on the skin*. The circuit is divided into twelve lines or meridians known

---

* refer also to the schematic time chart in the latter part of this book.

4

as Organ Meridians. There are also four pairs of Vessel Meridians not included in the circuit. In this work we shall be considering the Organ Meridians and only two of the Vessel Meridians as these last are closely allied to the Organ Meridians. The significance of the two Vessel Meridians PIII(i) and PIV(i) has not yet been adequately appreciated by Western writers on Acupuncture, these meridians will be treated more fully in some future volume. In this present work all the points on the two meridians PIII(i) and PIV(i) are enumerated and, where treatment is recommended on them they are included in the Repertory.

Each of the twelve Organ-Meridians (cutaneous lines) is intimately linked to one of the twelve internal organs. The twelve organs recognized in Chinese medicine are not all the same as those recognized in Western Medicine. These have been outlined in our previous work* to which reference should be made.

There are approximately eight hundred *known* points on the Meridians and, in addition to these, there is a number of special points not on the meridians. According to de la Fuÿe it is only necessary for a person to learn some three hundred of the points in order to become a good acupuncturist. In our previous book we gave sixty-four psychism points, but, as fifty-four of these are bilateral, the total is 118 (108 plus 10); those together with the present book should furnish ample material for most practical purposes. We have prepared diagrams illustrating the starting and finishing points of each of the Organ meridians and *approximately* indicated the paths; special diagrams illustrate exact locations of points listed for treatment. There is a reason for omitting detailed tracing of whole paths, which omission might at first appear serious.

Western writers suggest that one of the reasons put forward by opponents of Acupuncture is that the Meridians follow no paths known to western anatomists (e.g. nerves, arteries, zones, etc.). We believe that, on the contrary, if we look *in the right place* or *at the right level* a logical anatomical path can be found linking all the points on the meridians with their related internal organs. We feel that there must be a simple set of principles upon which the meridians were mapped out in the first place and that, once the appro-

---

* Chinese System of Healing, Health Science Press.

5

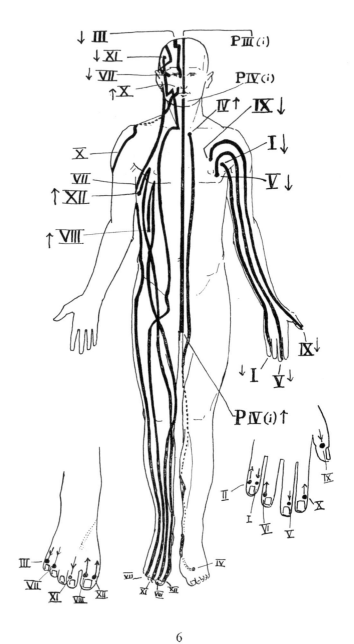

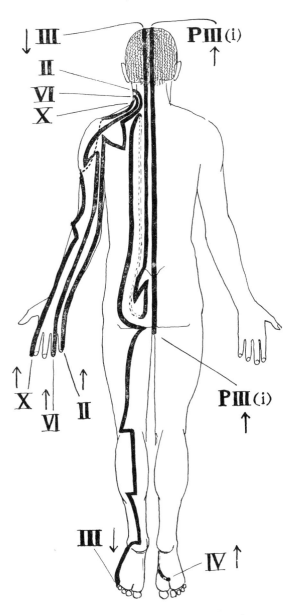

Front view and back view of human figure showing paths of the twelve Organ Meridians.

priate principles have been re-discovered, it should be possible to arrive at a sound reason for an exact anatomical positioning: such a re-discovery would be important in enabling one to settle, on logical grounds, differences in opinion among various 'authorities' regarding placing of some points. Furthermore when one comes across congenital structural deformities or abnormalities (e.g. six lumbar vertebrae instead of the usual five; eleven ribs instead of the usual twelve, etc.) or abnormalities due to injury, disease, or surgery it would then be possible to decide, with confidence based on application of sound principles, where, in each particular case, a point should be placed. We have already made considerable progress in this research, but it would be premature at this moment to publish ideas which might perhaps after fuller investigation prove to be erroneous.

Treatment at points can be either 'in tonification' or 'in sedation (dispersion)'. If there is not enough activity or tone the condition is said to be YIN, and stimulation (tonification) is required. If there is too much activity (hypertonicity) the condition is said to be YANG, and sedative (dispersion) action must be taken to restore balance.

How does one assess the patient's condition: is it YANG or is it YIN?

The question ever present in our mind would run something like this: Which of the forces is out of balance (in excess or deficiency) to bring about this condition, and at what places is the flow disturbed?

There would be a routine examination and questioning appearing very similar in many respects to traditional Western method. The Far-Eastern healer attaches great importance to the examination of the abdomen; he notes the tonicity of the abdominal musculature, any painful areas, shape, size, hardness, fluidity, and so on.*

Diagnosis and treatment through the manipulation of the abdomen is by no means limited to China; the Priest-doctors of

* Acupuncture et Médecine Chinoise vérifée au Japon, T. Nakayama, Paris 1934. ed. du Trianon.

Tibet have developed a highly specialized technique for what they refer to as "bloodless operation"**.

Examination of the patient will ordinarily include palpation of the Alarm Points (see diagram). These are points which, if spontaneously painful or painful under *light* digital pressure draw the practitioner's attention to an organ in more or less urgent need of attention. The Alarm point of an organ is not necessarily placed on that Organ Meridian. It will be noticed from the diagram that all the Alarm Points are on the anterior aspect of the trunk.

There are many signs by which a practitioner gleans indications of where derangement is likely to be found, not only through such signs as are familiar to homœopathic practitioners (colour of skin, texture of hair, look of the eyes, condition of finger nails, manner, posture, etc.), but through various blemishes, moles, beauty-spots, puckering of the skin, pimples, etc., etc. As for example:

A mole at the wing of the nose may indicate chronic or congenital tendency to Large Intestine disturbance, whereas a pustule or other transient blemish at the same point (X.20) would indicate acute derangement.

A blemish on the lobule of the ear often indicates Small Intestine derangement, chronic or acute according to the nature of the blemish (chilblain, eczema, pimple, mole, etc.). The traditional 'gipsy' remedy, for certain illnesses, of piercing at this point (11.19) and the wearing of silver or gold earrings may well have originated in China!

A blemish on the tragus (VII.2) will tend to relate to Gall Bladder derangement: a blemish at the point on the helix just below the level of the zygomatic arch (VI.23) indicates the Thermo-Regulator (Three-Heater) System; as would also eczema or other blemish near the mastoid process (VI.17).

The point just below the internal angle of the orbital cavity at the root of the nose (III.1) or on the superciliary eminence (III.2) will serve as good indications of chronic or acute affections of the Bladder.

* Tibetische Medizinphilosophie. P. Cyrill v Korvin-Krasinski. Origo Verlag. Zürich 1953.

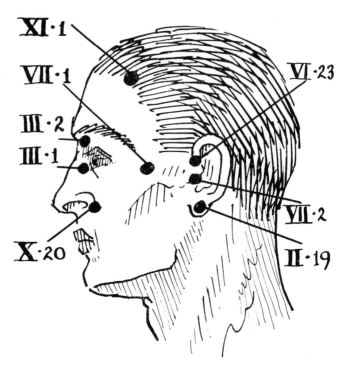

Side view of the head showing
X.20 II.19, VII.2, V1.23 & VI.17

It should further be noted that a particular malady or defect may well have its positive or negative polarity. For example: — In Faber's Medical Dictionary*, Myopia is described as: "An anomaly of optical refraction in which focal images from parallel

rays are formed in front of the retina *either* owing to too great a length of the visual axis *or* to an increase in curvature or refractory power of the ocular media." The former is a YIN condition and the latter a YANG condition.

Stammering may be due to spasmodic *contraction* of throat musculature, a YANG condition, or it might be due to an uncon-

* edited by Sir Cecil Wakeley, Bt., Faber and Faber Limited. London 1953 edition.

10

trolled flow with constant repetition of some sounds, the words not being confined nor sounds kept within bounds—, a YIN condition.

The Chinese Pulses, however, can be considered as *the* characteristic diagnostic method. Through feeling the pulses (note the plural) the practitioner assesses the condition of any organ or any part of the body, including psycho-logical states. The pulses technique has been developed over many centuries.

Some authorities consider that a working knowledge of the Chinese pulses is absolutely essential if one wishes to become an efficient practitioner; others seem to feel that it is not essential for, they say, if the indications given by the pulses conflict with assessment arrived at by other clinical examination, the verdict of the pulses should be ignored.

Our own view is that ability to take the Chinese pulses and rely on them as a principal diagnostic requires a great deal of experience combined with a high degree of natural sensitivity, intuition and faith. We do, nevertheless, feel that through the radial pulses, without necessarily using any other diagnostic technique, a patient's needs can be adequately assessed.

In Chinese medicine there are fourteen radial pulses (on the radial artery at the wrist). There are also nine peripheral pulses, which are simple alternative points at which nine of the radial pulses can be felt.

As will be seen from the illustration, there are three positions on each wrist. On the left wrist at each of these three positions two pulses are distinguished, one superficial and one deep. On the right wrist, at position One, two pulses are to be felt, a superficial and a deep; but at position Two and Three the pulses are felt at three levels, superficial, middle, and deep.

The photograph illustration shows how the fingers should be placed in order to take the pulses. Before taking the pulses the patient should be recumbent, relaxed and quiet for at least half an hour. Pulses on the right wrist are felt with the fingers of the right hand; pulses on the left wrist are taken with the fingers of the left

11

hand. (Although Stiefvater, on page 26 (Akupunktur als Neural-therapie) gives these instructions in the text, his illustration on page 24 shows the pulses of the right hand being palpated with the fingers of the left hand)

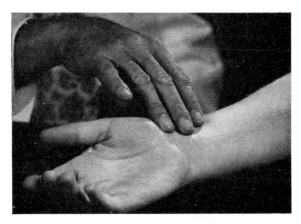

Photograph showing technique for taking pulse

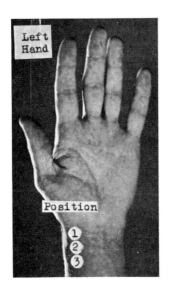 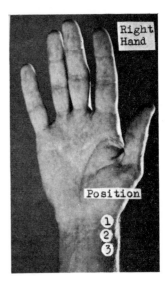

Photograph of hands showing Positions of pulses

The exact positions are found by first placing the middle finger on the middle of the apophysis of the radius, the first and ring fingers then fall naturally into the correct positions. The first finger will be in the small hollow on the proximal side of the apophysis; and the ring finger at the base of the thumb, just proximal to the thenar eminence. (*see illustration*). The pulse is felt with the pad of the finger (last phalange) lightly rested in position for the superficial pulse; and pressed heavily for the deep pulse, not so heavily, of course, as to crush the artery against the bone. On the right wrist where the pulse is taken at three levels, the pressure must be delicately adjusted to light, medium, and heavy pressure.

The practitioner represents the state of the pulse by assigning a number from 0 to 8. 4 represents Normal, 3 to 0 represents a YIN condition, 5 to 8 represents a YANG condition. *Any* departure from Normal (4) indicates that the organ associated with that pulse is deranged or troubled *to some degree* and requires treatment either in tonification or in sedation.

According to Dr. de la Füÿe, a relatively little experience suffices to enable one to recognize a YIN or a YANG condition, but it takes a long experience to be able to form a clear picture of the illness and to assess the exact points to be treated, for one needs to distinguish subtleties of width, length, form, movement, and placing of the pulse*.

* Dr. de la Fuye, in a lecture given to students of Acupuncture and circulated to them in duplicated form, gives pulse diagnosis in considerable detail; we hope this paper will one day be translated into English and made available to English speaking people.

Dr. Stiefvater's simplification of pulse interpretation should, however, enable a practitioner to make a sound beginning in the general assessment of YIN or YANG conditions:—

"Small, thin, fine: Insufficiency.

Full and hard: Hypertension, Hyperfunction.

Soft and strong: Inflammation.

Small, hard and pointed: Spasticity, contractures, usually an organ painful.

Overflowing and large: Excess, usually with inflammation and pain.

Very weak, scarcely perceptible: Energy depletion."**

**pages 26 of 1956 edition Akupunktur als Neuraltherapie.

If treatment at a particular point is appropriate that point will tend to be more or less painful under digital pressure, or it may even be spontaneously painful, whereas on a healthy person such point is not normally painful.* This is not always the case for there are

* As an illustrative example: A friend wrote a despairing letter, saying that his wife was still putting on weight alarmingly in spite of having tried dozens of different treatments. Our friend wondered whether we could suggest anything to try. We knew him to be a keen homœopathist; so we gave a list of twelve points at which obesity would ordinarily be treated by acupuncture, and their homœopathic remedy correspondencies, suggesting that he palpate each of these points, some of which would probably be painful under pressure. We told him, further, that he could then either massage these points in the Chinese way or himself prescribe remedies in potency guided by these indications. About four days later we had a letter back from him to the effect that he had tested all these points on his wife and on himself. On her 8 of the points were very painful under pressure; on him *not one* of them was painful, not even under fairly heavy digital pressure.

times when a point may be treated *in anticipation*: for example, X.1 may be treated in sedation (silver needle) prior to a tooth extraction (Soulie de Morant).

> *Anticipatory or Preventive Treatment using the* FIVE ELEMENTS METHOD *will be the subject of another work, now in preparation.*

The careful checking of Point and Potency Remedy correspondencies has been carried out clinically over many years by Dr. de la Fuÿe, who has verified or amended many of the "Weihe"* points.

* Die Weihische Schmerzpunktmethode, Drs. Weihe & Göhrum, Leipzig 1903.

The "relatively little experience" referred to on page 14, however, should be based upon a thorough understanding of the YIN-YANG Science principles. In our view the minimum requirement is that the Unique Principle of FOU-HI and his twelve propositions should be learned and *understood,* since these form the basis from which all else is deducible.

In an Appendix we quote from Dr. Nyoiti Sakurazawa's PRINCIPE UNIQUE de la Philosophie et de la Science d'Extrême-Orient (Vrin 1958), together with our translation.

AL

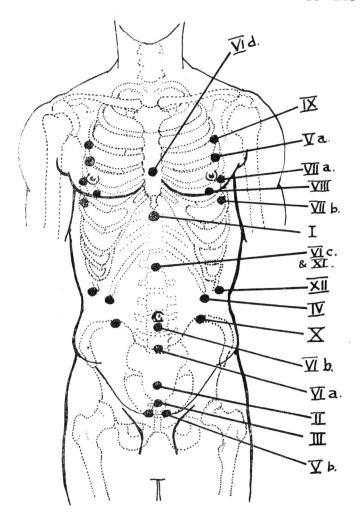

VI d.

IX

V a.

VII a.

VIII

VII b.

I

VI c.
& XI.

XII

IV

X

VI b.

VI a.

II

III

V b.

ALARM POINTS

15

I.

The Alarm Point of meridian I (Heart) is at PIV(i).14

Anatomical position: Median: at the junction of the superior quarter and middle quarter of a line drawn from the xiphoid process to the umbilicus. Also called the Solar Plexus point.

Spontaneous pain at this point indicates a gastro-cardiac disorder.

Polarity of Treatment: Sedative, needle 2—4 mm.

Homœopathic remedy: IPECA 6 — 12 (Weihe)

Tabacum 12 — 30 (de la Fuye)

II.

The Alarm Point of meridian II (Small Intestine) is at PIV(i).4

Anatomical position: Median: at the junction of the middle and lower third of a line drawn from the umbilicus to the superior border of the pubis symphisis.

Spontaneous pain at this point indicates disorder of the small intestine.

Polarity of Treatment: Tonification or Sedative, needle 5 — 25 mm.

Homœopathic remedy: HYDRASTIS 6 — 30 (Weihe).

III.

The Alarm Point of meridian III (Bladder) is at PIV(i).3

Anatomical position: Median: 4 cm superior to the pubis symphisis. Spontaneous pain at this point indicates bladder disorder.

16

Polarity of Treatment: Sedative, needle 2 mm — 2 cm.

Homœopathic Remedy: RHUS TOX 3 — 12 (Weihe)

IV.

The Alarm Point of meridian IV (Kidneys) is at VII.25

Anatomical Position: Bilateral: at the free end of the twelfth rib.

Spontaneous pain at this point indicates Kidney disorder with associated Gall bladder trouble.

Polarity of Treatment: Sedative, needle 2 — 5 mm.

Homœopathic remedy: BERBERIS 3x — 12 de la Fuye.

V.

There are two Alarm Points of meridian V (Circulation—Sexfield) (a) at V.1, and (b) at IV.11

(a)

Anatomical position: Bilateral; on the anterior face of the fourth rib, 2 cm beyond the external rim of the mamelonary areola (2 cm outside medioclavicular line).

Polarity of Treatment: Sedative, needle 2 mm — 1 cm

Homœopathic remedy: CACTUS 6 (Weihe, left side: de lay Fuye, right side)

(b)

Anatomical position: Bilateral: 4 cm from the centre line of the pubis symphisis, almost on the superior border of the os pubis. Stiefvater places it at 2 cm.

Polarity of Treatment: Tonification or Sedative, needle 2 mm — 1 cm.

Homœopathic remedy: CANTHARIS 6 — 30 (de la Fuye)

VI

There are four Alarm Points of this meridian (Three-Heater) placed at PIV(i) .5, .7, .12, & .17

(a) at PIV(i) .5

Anatomical position: Median: at the junction of the upper quarter and lower three quarters of a line drawn from the umbilicus to the pubis symphisis.

Polarity of Treatment: Sedative, needle 2 mm — 2 cm.

Homœopathic remedy: PHOSPHORUS 6—30 (de la Fuÿe)

(b) at PIV(i) .7

Anatomical position: Median: 2 cm below the umbilicus.

Polarity of Treatment: Sedative, needle 4 mm — 2 cm.

Homœopathic remedy: CANTHARIS 6—200 (de la Fuÿe)

(c) at PIV(i) .12

Anatomical position: Median: 1 cm above the mid-point of a line drawn from the umbilicus to the xiphoid process (at the level of the sterno-costal angle).

Polarity of Treatment: Sedative, needle 2 mm — 2 cm.

Homœopathic remedy: THUYA 6 — 200 (Weihe)

(d) at PIV(i) .17

Anatomical position: Median: on the sternum at the level of the fourth inter-costal space.

Polarity of Treatment: Sedative, needle 1 mm — 6 mm.

Homœopathic remedy: RAPHANUS SATIVUS 6 (Weihe).

VII

The two Alarm Points for meridian VII (Gall Bladder) are at VII .23 & .24

(a) at VII .23

Anatomical position: Bilateral: in the fifth inter-costal space on the anterior paraxillary line of Weihe.

Polarity of Treatment: Sedative, needle 2 mm—6 mm.

Homœopathic remedy: CHELIDONIUM 3x—30 (de la Fuÿe)

18

(b) at VII .24

Anatomical position: Bilateral: in the sixth inter-costal space, on
the anterior paraxillary line of Weihe.

Polarity of Treatment: Sedative, 2 mm—6 mm.

Homœopathic remedy: KALI CARB 6—30 (de la Fuÿe)

VIII

The Alarm Point of meridian VIII (Liver) is at VIII .14

Anatomical Position: Bilateral: below the nipple in the fifth inter-
costal space.

Polarity of Treatment: Sedative, needle 2 mm—6 mm.

Homœopathic remedy: NUX MOSCHATA 30 (Weihe).

IX

The Alarm Point of meridian IX (Lungs) is at IX.1

Anatomical position: Bilateral: in the third inter-costal space on
the anterior paraxillary line of Weihe.

Polarity of Treatment: Sedative, needle 2 mm—6 mm.

Homœopathic remedy: HEPAR SULF 6 (Weihe, right side, de la
Fuÿe, left side).

X.

The Alarm Point of meridian X (Large Intestine) is at XI .25

Anatomical position: Bilateral: 6 cm lateral to the umbilicus.

Polarity of Treatment: Sedative, needle 2 mm—2 cm.

Homœopathic remedy: right side BERBERIS 6—30 (Weihe)
left side SEPIA 30 (Weihe)

XI

The Alarm Point of meridian XI (Stomach) is at the same point as Alarm of meridian VI, (c).

XII

The Alarm Point of meridian XII (Spleen-Pancreas) is at XII.15

Anatomical position: Bilateral; at the free end of the eleventh rib.

Polarity of Treatment: Sedative, needle 3 mm—1 cm.

Homœopathic remedy: NUX VOMICA 6—30 (Weihe) right side
CHINA 6—30 (Weihe) left side
CEANOTHUS 6—30 (Weihe) left side

MERIDIAN POINTS

The Points on the Organ Meridians are arranged in the following groups:

Toning Points (TN)
Sedative Points (SD)
Regulator Points (RG)
Passage Points (PS)
Vesicular Re-inforcement Points (VR)

each group is subdivided into the following: —

points on the three Centrifugal YIN   organ meridians
points on the three Centripetal YANG organ meridians
points on the three Centrifugal YANG organ meridians
points on the three Centripetal YIN   organ meridians

Toning Points of meridians I. V. & IX.

I.

The principal toning point on meridian I (Heart) is at I.9

Anatomical position: Bilateral: on the dorsum of the hand, on the last phalange of the little finger, 2 mm above and exterior to the external ungueal angle (thumb side).

Polarity of Treatment: Tonification, needle 1 mm—2 mm

Homœopathic remedy: DIGITALIS 6 (de la Fuÿe)

V.

The principal toning point on meridian V (Circulation—Sexfield) is at V.9

Anatomical position: Bilateral: on the dorsum of the hand, on the last phalange of the middle finger, 2 mm above and exterior to the external ungueal angle (thumb side).

Polarity of Treatment: Tonification, needle 1 mm—2 mm

Homœopathic remedy: ACONITUM 1—3 (de la Fuÿe)
GINSENG 1—3 (de la Fuÿe)

IX.

The principal toning point on meridian IX (Lungs) is at IX.9

Anatomical position: Bilateral: on the anterior of the wrist on the radial groove at the wrist-fold (antero-inferior of the tendon of the supinator longus).

Polarity of Treatment: Tonification, needle 2 mm—5 mm.

Homœopathic remedy: AMMON CARB 3—6 (de la Fuÿe)

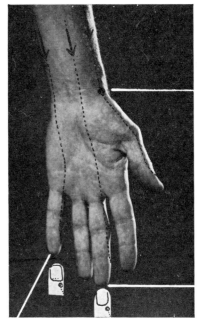

IX.9   TRAE-IUANN
ammon. carb 3—6
(de la Fuÿe)
2—5 mm

V.9 TCHONG-TCHRONG
aconitum 1—3
ginseng 1—3
(de la Fuÿe)
1—2 mm.

I.9   CHAO-TCHRONG
digitalis 6 (de la Fuÿe), 1—2 mm.

The Principal bilateral Toning point (TN) on each of the three Centrifugal YIN Organ Meridians:

I.   HEART
V.   CIRCULATION—SEXFIELD
IX.   LUNGS

23

II.

The principal toning point on meridian II (Small intestine) is at II.3

Anatomical position: Bilateral: on the ulnar side of the hand, about 2 cm above the metacarpo-phalangeal articulation of the little finger.

Polarity of Treatment: Tonification, needle 2 mm—6 mm.
Homœopathic remedy: PLUMBUM 30—200 (de la Fuÿe)

VI.

The principal tonining point on meridian VI (Three-Heater or Thermo-Regulator) is at VI.3

Anatomical position: Bilateral: on the dorsum of the hand, between the upper extremities of the fourth and fifth metacarpals, about 4 cm below the inferior ulnar apophysis.

Polarity of Treatment: Tonification, needle 2 mm—6 mm.

Homœopathic Remedy: SILICEA 30—M (de la Fuÿe)

X.

The principal toning point on meridian X (Large intestine) is at X.11

Anatomical position: Bilateral: on the antero-extern of the elbow, exactly at the extremity of the elbow-fold in hyperflexion.

Polarity of Treatment: Tonification, needle 2 mm—1 cm.

Homœopathic remedy: ALUMINA 30 (de la Fuÿe).

X.11 TSIOU-TCHRE
alumina 30
(de la Fuÿe)
2 mm.—1 cm.

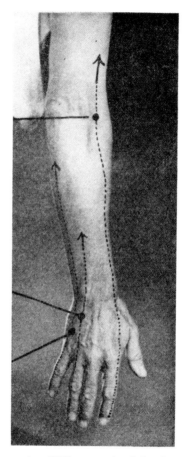

VI.3 TCHONG-TCHOU
silicea 30—M
(de la Fuÿe)
2—6 mm.

II.3 REOU-TSRI
plumbum 30—200
(de la Fuÿe)
2—6 mm.

The Principal bilateral Toning point (TN) on each of the three Centripetal YANG Organ Meridians:

II.   Small Intestine
VI.   Thermo-Regulator or Three Heater
X.   Large Intestine

Toning Points of meridians III. VII. & XI.

III.

The principal toning point on meridian III (Bladder) is at III.67

Anatomical position: Bilateral: on the dorsal surface of the fifth toe, on the last phalange, 2 mm proximal and lateral to the external ungueal angle.

Polarity of Treatment: Tonification, needle 1—2 mm.

Homœopathic remedy: KALI CARB 3x—12 (de la Fuÿe)

VII.

The principal toning point on meridian VII (Gall bladder) is at VII.43

Anatomical position: Bilateral: on the dorsum of the foot, lateral base of the fourth toe.

Polarity of Treatment: Tonification, needle 2—6 mm

Homœopathic remedy: CHINA 6 (de la Fuÿe)

XI.

The principal toning point on meridian XI (Stomach) is at XI.41

Anatomical position: Bilateral: on the dorsum of the foot, above the scaphoid & cuboid, below the tibia.

Polarity of Treatment: Tonification, needle 2 mm—10 mm.

Homœopathic remedy: GRAPHITES 3x—6x (de la Fuÿe)

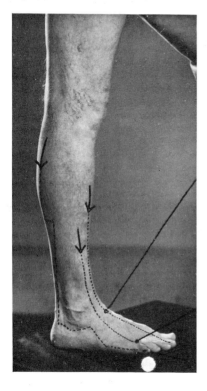

XI.41   TSIE-TSRI
graphites 3x—6x
(de la Fuÿe)
2—10 mm.

VII.43   SIE-TSRI
china 6   (de la Fuÿe)
2—6 mm.

III.67   TCHE-INN
kali carb. 3x—12
1—2 mm.   (de la Fuÿe)

The Principal bilateral Toning Points (TN) on each of the three
Centrifugal YANG Organ Meridians:

III.   Bladder
VII.   Gall Bladder
XII.   Stomach

27

Toning Points of meridians IV, VIII. & XII.

IV.

The principal toning point on meridian IV (Kidneys) is at IV.7

Anatomical position: Bilateral; about 6 cm above the internal malleolus, and 1 cm posterior to the tibia.

Polarity of Treatment: Tonification, needle 2 mm—6 mm.

Homœopathic remedy: SEPIA 6—30 (de la Fuÿe)
MERC. SOL 6—30 (de la Fuÿe)

VIII.

The principal toning point on meridian VIII (Liver) is at VIII.9

Anatomical position: Bilateral: on the internal aspect of the flexed knee, at the extremity of the transverse fold.

Polarity of Treatment: Tonification, needle 2 mm—1 cm.

Homœopathic remedy: LYCOPODIUM 12—30 (de la Fuÿe)

XII.

The principal toning point on meridian XII (Spleen-Pancreas is at XII.2

Anatomical position: Bilateral: on the internal surface of the big toe, just distal to the metatarso-phalangeal articulation.

Polarity of Treatment: Tonification, needle 2 mm—6 mm.

Homœopathic remedy: ARSEN ALB 6—30 (de la Fuÿe)

Toning points

IV, VIII, XII

VIII.9 TSIOU-TSIUANN
   lycopodium 12—30
                (de la Fuÿe)
   2 mm.—1 cm.

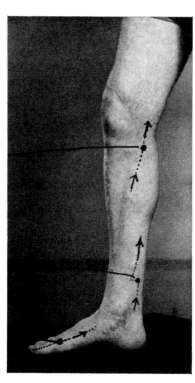

IV.7 FOU-LEOU
   sepia 6—30
   merc. sol. 6—30
                (de la Fuÿe)
   2—6 mm.

XII.2 TA-TOU
   arsen. alb. 6—30
                (de la Fuÿe)
   2—6 mm.

The Principal bilateral Toning Points (TN) on each of the three Centripetal YIN Organ Meridians

      IV.   Kidneys
   VIII.   Liver
   XII.   Spleen—Pancreas

Sedative Points of meridians I. V. & IX.

I.

The principal sedative point on meridian I (Heart) is at I.7

Anatomical position: Bilateral: on the palmar surface of the hand on the hypothenar eminence at the anterior external border of the pisiform.

Polarity of Treatment: Sedative, needle 2 mm—9 mm.

Homœopathic remedy: AURUM MET 30—200 (de la Fuÿe)
                        SPIGELIA   3x— 12 (de la Fuÿe)

V.

The principal sedative point on meridian V (Circulation—Sexfield) is at V.7

Anatomical position: Bilateral; on the anterior of the wrist, on the centre of the lunate.

Polarity of Treatment: Sedative, needle 2 mm—1 cm.

Homœopathic remedies:

           Circulation SPIGELIA   3— 6 (de la Fuÿe)
           Sexfield STAPHYSAGRIA 6—30 (de la Fuÿe)
                   MUREX   30 (de la Fuÿe)
              ORIGANUM   6 (de la Fuÿe)

IX.

The principal sedative point on meridian IX (Lungs) is at IX.5

Anatomical position: Bilateral: in the middle of the elbow fold.

Polarity of Treatment: Sedative, needle 2 mm—1 cm.

Homœopathic remedy: FERRUM PHOS   6—30 (de la Fuÿe)
                     AGARICUS   6—30 (de la Fuÿe)

SD

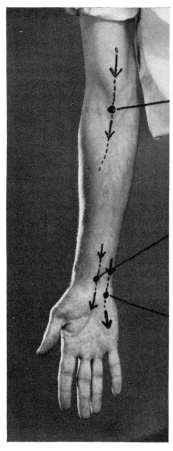

IX.5 TCHRE-TSRE
ferrum phos 6—12
(de la Fuÿe)
2 mm—1 cm.

V.7 TA-LING
circulation
spigellia 3—6
sex-field
m. Staphysagria 6—30
f. murex 30
origanum 6
(de la Fuÿe)
needle
2 mm—1 cm.

I.7 CHENN-MENN
aurum met. 30—200
spigelia 3x—12
(de la Fuÿe)
2—9 mm.

The Principal bilateral Sedative point (SD) on each of the three Centrifugal YIN Organ Meridians

    I. Heart
    V. Circulation—Sexfield
  IX. Lungs

II.

The principal sedative point of meridian II (Small intestine) is at II.8

Anatomical position: Bilateral: Postero-internal of the elbow, inferior internal of olecranon fossa.

Polarity of Treatment: Sedative, needle 2 mm—5 mm.

Homœopathic remedy: OENANTHE CROCATA 6—30 (de la Fuÿe)

VI.

The principal sedative point of meridian VI (Three-Heater) is at VI.10

Anatomical position: Bilateral: in the olecranon fossa, 1 cm above the centre of the olecranon (on the triceps tendon).

Polarity of Treatment: Sedative, needle 2 mm—1 cm.

Homœopathic remedy: PHOSPHORUS 6—30 (de la Fuÿe)

X.

The principal sedative points of meridian X (Large Intestine) are at X.2 & X.3

NOTE: *These two points must be treated simultaneously*

Anatomical positions: Bilateral: .2 is just below, and .3 is just above the metacarpo-phalangeal articulation on the index finger (thumb side).

Polarity of Treatment: Sedative, needle 2 mm—5 mm.

Homœopathic remedy: ARGENTUM NITRICUM 6 (de la Fuÿe)

SD

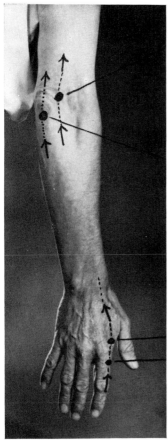

VI.10 TIENN-TSING
phosphorus 6—30
(de la Fuÿe)
2 mm—1 cm.

II.8 SIAO-RAE
Oenanthe crocata 6—-30
(de la Fuÿe)
2—5 mm.

X.2 & .3 EL-TSIENN &
SANN-TSIENN
argentum nitricum 6
(de la Fuÿe)
2—5 mm.
Note both these points must be
treated simultaneously

The Principal bilateral Sedative Points (SD) on each of the three
Centripetal YANG Organ Meridians

    II.   Small Intestine
   VI.   Thermo-Regulator or Three-Heater
    X.   Large Intestine

33

Sedative points of meridians III. VII. & XI.

III.

The principal sedative point of meridian III (Bladder) is at III.65

Anatomical position: Bilateral: on the external aspect of the foot, just behind the metatarso-phalangeal articulation of the little toe, below the fifth metatarsal.

Polarity of Treatment: Sedative, needle 2 mm—6 mm.

Homœopathic remedies: CANTHARIS 6   (de la Fuÿe)
                        NUX VOMICA 6—30 (de la Fuÿe)

VII.

The principal sedative point of meridian VII (Gall-bladder) is at VII.38

Anatomical position: Bilateral: on the antero-external aspect of the leg, 10 cm above the external malleolus, on the line drawn from the external malleolus to the external border of the anterior tuberosity of the tibia.

Polarity of Treatment: Sedative, needle 2 mm—2 cm.

Homœopathic remedy: BERBERIS 3—6 (de la Fuÿe)

XI.

The principal sedative point of meridian XI (Stomach) is at XI.45

Anatomical position: Bilateral: on the dorsum of the foot, second toe, 2 mm above and exterior to the external ungueal angle.

Polarity of Treatment: Sedative, needle 1 mm—4 mm.

Homœopathic remedy: NUX VOMICA 6—12 (de la Fuÿe)

VII.38 IANG-FOU
 berberis 3x—6
  (de la Fuÿe)
 2 mm.—2 cm.

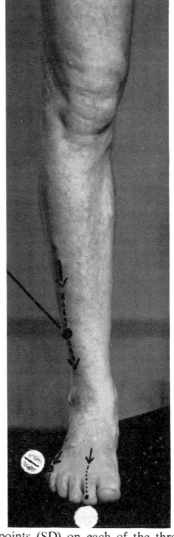

III.65 CHOU-KOU
 cantharis 6
 nux vomica 6—30
  (de la Fuÿe)
 2—6 mm.

XI.45 LI-TOE
 nux vomica 6—12
  (de la Fuÿe)
 1—4 mm.

The Principal bilateral Sedative points (SD) on each of the three Centrifugal YANG Organ Meridians:

　　 III. Bladder
　　 VII. Gall-Bladder
　　 XI. Stomach

Sedative points of meridians IV. VIII. & XII.

IV.

The principal sedative points on meridian IV (Kidneys) are at
IV.1 & 2

IV.1

Anatomical position: Bilateral: on the sole of the foot, between the two pads at the base of the first and other toes.

Polarity of Treatment: Sedative, needle 2 mm—1 cm.

Homœopathic remedy: LYCOPODIUM 6—12 (de la Füye)

IV.2

Anatomical position: Bilateral: just below the scaphoid prominence.

Polarity of Treatment: Sedative, needle 2 mm—6 mm.

Homœopathic remedy: SULPHUR 30—200 (de la Füye)

VIII.

The principal sedative point on meridian VIII (Liver) is at VIII.2

Anatomical position: Bilateral: on the dorsum of the foot, in the space between the first and second toes towards the base of the first toe.

Polarity of Treatment: Sedative, needle 1 mm—5 mm.

Homœopathic remedy: BRYONY 3—6 (de la Füye)

XII.

The principal sedative point on meridian XII (Spleen-Pancreas) is at XII.5

Anatomical position: Bilateral: about 4 cm below and in front of the internal malleolus, in the hollow between the navicular and cuneiform.

Polarity of Treatment: Sedative, needle 2 mm—6 mm.

Homœopathic remedy: SILICEA 30—200 (de la Füye)
FLUORICUM ACIDUM 12—30
(de la Füye)

SD

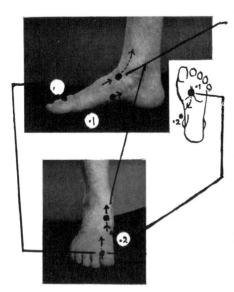

XII.5
  CHANG-TSIOU
silicea 30—200
fluoricum acidum
            12—30
      (de la Fuÿe)
2—6 mm.

—IV.1
IONG-TS'IUANN
lycopodium 6—12
      (de la Fuÿe)
2 mm—1 cm.
IV.2 JENN-KOU
sulphur 30—200
      (de la Fuÿe)
2—6 mm.

VIII.2 SING-TSIENN
bryonia 3—6
1—5 mm.
      (de la Fuÿe)

The Principal bilateral Sedative points (SD) on each of the three Centripetal YIN Organ Meridians:

IV.   Kidneys
VIII.   Liver
XII.   Spleen—Pancreas

37

Regulator points on meridians I. V. & IX.

I.

The Regulator point (hypertonifying and hypersedative) on meridian I (Heart) is at the same position as the principal sedative point, I.7

Anatomical position: As Sedative point, q.v.

Homœopathic remedies:
    Hypersedative: ACONITUM 6—30 (de la Fuÿe)
    Hypertonification: CRATAEGUS TM—3x (de la Fuÿe)

V.

The Regulator point (hypertonifying and hypersedative) on meridian V (Circulation—Sexfield) is at the same position as the principal sedative point, V.7

Anatomical position: As Sedative point, q.v.

Homœopathic remedies:
    Hypersedative: CACTUS 6 (de la Fuÿe)
        males STAPHYSAGRIA 200—DM
            (de la Fuÿe)
        females MUREX 200 (de la Fuÿe)
        ORIGANUM 30 (de la Fue)

    Hypertonifying: NAJA 6 (de la Fuÿe)
        GINSENG TM, 10 drops per day
            (de la Fuÿe)

IX.

The Regulator point (hypertonifying and hypersedative) on meridian IX (Lungs) is at the same position as the principal toning point, IX.9

Anatomical position: As Toning point, q.v.

Homœopathic remedies:
    Hypersedative: SANGUINARIA 6 (de la Fuÿe)
    Hypertonifying: CARBO VEG 6—30 (de la Fuÿe)

RG

Regulator points

I, V, IX.

IX.9 TRAE-IUANN
Hyperton: carbo veg. 6—30
Hypersed: sanguinaria 6
(de la Fuÿe)
2 mm—1 cm.

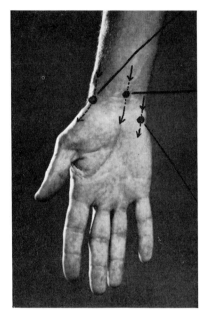

V.7 TA-LING
Hyperton:
naja 6
gingseng TM
Hypersed:
cactus 6
m. staphysagria
200—DM
f. murex 200
origanum 30
(de la Fuÿe)
2 mm—1 cm.

I.7 CHENN-MENN
Hyperton:
cratoegus TM—3x
Hypersed:
aconitum 6—30
(de la Fuÿe)
2—9 mm.

The bilateral Regulator (RG) points, hypertonifying and hypersedative on each of the three Centrifugal YIN Organ Meridians:

I.   Heart
V.   Circulation—Sexfield
IX. Lungs

Regulator points on meridians II. VI. & X.

II.

The Regulator point (hypertonifying and hypersedative) on meridian II (small intestine) is at II.4

Anatomical position: Bilateral: on the ulna border of the hand, 2 cm below the wrist fold, on the internal aspect of the base of the fifth metacarpal.

Homœopathic remedies:

    Hypersedative: CUPRUM MET 30—200 (de la Fuÿe) reinforces action at II.3
    needle 2 mm—10 mm.

    Hypertonifying: ALUMINA 6—30 (de la Fuÿe) reinforces action at II.3
    needle 2 mm—10 mm.

VI.

The Regulator point (hypertonifying and hypersedative) on meridian VI (Three-Heater) is at VI.4

Anatomical position: Bilateral: on the dorsum of the wrist in the articular line of the hamate and fourth metacarpal.

Homœopathic remedies:

    Hypersedative: SULPHUR 30—M (de la Fuÿe) reinforces action at VI.10
    needle 2 mm—6 mm

    Hypertonifying: PSORINUM 30—M (de la Fuÿe) reinforces action at VI.3
    needle 2 mm—6 mm

X.

The Regulator point (hypertonifying and hypersedative) on meridian X (large intestine) is at X.4

Anatomical position: Bilateral: on the dorsum of the hand, in the angle formed by the first and second metacarpals.

Homœopathic remedies:

    Hypersedative: VERAT ALB 6 (de la Fuÿe) reinforces action at X.2 & .3
    needle 2 mm—4 mm (de la Fuÿe)
    .5—2 cm (Stiefvater)

    Hypertonifying: OPIUM 30—M (de la Fuÿe)
    HYDRASTIS 6 (de la Fuÿe) reinforces action at X.11

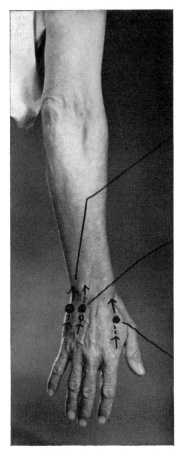

II.4 OANN-KOU
  Hyperton: alumina 6—30
  Hypersed: cuprum met
    (de la Fuye)
                     30—200
  2—10 mm.

VI.4 IANG—TCHRE
  Hyperton: psorinum
                  30—200—M
  Hypersed: sulphur
                  30—200—M
    (de la Fuÿe)
  2—6 mm.

X.4 RO-KOU
  Hyperton: opium 30—M
  Hyperton: hydrastis 6
  Hypersed: verat. alb. 6
    (de la Fuÿe)
  2—4 mm. (de la Fuÿe)
  .5—2 cm. (Stiefvater)

The bilateral Regulator (RG) points, hypertonifying and hyper-sedative, on each of the three Centripetal YANG Organ Meridians:
    II.   Small Intestine
    XI.   Thermo-Regulator or Three-Heater
    X.   Large Intestine

Regulator points on meridians III. VII. & XI.

III.

The Regulator point (hypertonifying and hypersedative) on meridian III (Bladder) is at III.64

Anatomical position: Bilateral: on the external border of the foot, under the tubercle of the fifth metatarsal.

Homœopathic remedies:

Hypersedative: APIS 6—30 (de la Fuÿe)
reinforces action at III.65
needle 2 mm—6 mm.

Hypertonifying: CAUSTICUM 30 (de la Fuÿe)
reinforces action at III.67

VII.

The Regulator point (hypertonifying and hypersedative) on meridian VII (Gall bladder) is at VII.40

Anatomical position: Bilateral: on the antero-external aspect of the foot (instep) in the centre of the calcaneo-cuboid articulation.

Homœopathic remedies

Hypersedative: COLOCYNTHIS 6 (de la Fuÿe)
reinforces action at VII.38
needle 2—6 mm

Hypertonifying: LYCOPODIUM 6—12 (de la Fuÿe)
reinforces action at VII.43

XI.

The Regulator point (hypertonifying and hypersedative) on meridian XI (Stomach) is at XI.42

Anatomical position: Bilateral: on the dorsum of the foot (instep) at the meeting of the scaphoid and the second and third cuniforms.

Homœopathic remedies:

Hypersedative: NITRIC ACID 6 (de la Fuÿe)
reinforces action at XI.45
needle 2 mm—5 mm

Hypertonifying: ARSEN ALB 6—12 (de la Fuÿe)
reinforces action at XI.41

RG

Regulator points

III, VII, XI.

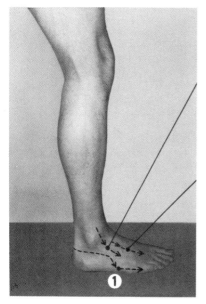

XI.42   TCHRONG-IANG
Hyperton:
  Arsen. alb. 6—12
Hypersed: Nitric acid 6
    (de la Fuÿe)
2—5 mm.

VII.40   TSIOU-SIU
Hyperton:
  Lycopodium 6—12
Hypersed: Colocynthis 6
    (de la Fuÿe)
2—6 mm.

III.64 TSING-KOU
Hyperton: Causticum 30
Hypersed: Apis 6—30
    (de la Fuÿe)
2—6 mm.

The bilateral Regulator points, hypertonifying and hyper-sedative, on each of the three Centrifugal YANG meridians:

 III. Bladder
 VII. Gall-Bladder
 XI. Stomach

Regulator points on meridians IV. VIII. & XII.

IV.

The regulator point (hypertonifying and hypersedative) on meridian
IV (Kidneys) is at IV.3

Anatomical position: Bilateral: on the internal aspect of the foot,
1 cm below and behind the internal malleolus

Homœopathic remedies:

Hypersedative: PHOSPHORUS 6—30 (de la Fuÿe)
reinforces action at IV.1 & .2
needle 2—6 mm.

Hypertonifying: ARSEN ALB 6—12 (de la Fuÿe)
reinforces action at IV.7

VIII.

The Regulator point (hypertonifying and hypersedative) on meridian
VIII (Liver) is at VIII.3

Anatomical position: Bilateral: on the anterior of the instep,
between the first and second metatarsals, a
little in front of their articulation with the
first cuniform.

Homœopathic remedies:

Hypersedative: CUPRUM MET 6—30 (de la Fuÿe)
reinforces action at VIII.2
needle 1 mm—5 mm

Hypertonifying: PHOSPHORUS 200—M (de la Fuÿe)
reinforces action at VIII.9

XII.

The Regulator point (hypertonifying and hypersedative) on meridian
XII (Spleen-Pancreas) is at XII.3

Anatomical position: Bilateral: on the internal aspect of the foot,
below and behind the metatarso-phalangeal
articulation of the big toe.

Homœopathic remedies:

Hypersedative: ALOE 6—30 (de la Fuÿe)
reinforces action at XII.5
needle 2 mm—6 mm.

Hypertonifying: CHINA 6 (de la Fuÿe)
reinforces action at XII.2

RG

Regulator points

IV, VIII, XII.

IV.3 TRAE-TSRI
Hyperton:
    Arsen alb. 6—12
Hypersed:
    Phosphorus 6—30
            (de la Fuÿe)
2—6 mm.

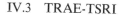

XII.3 TRAE-PO
Hyperton: China 6
Hypersed: Aloe 6—30
            (de la Fuÿe)
2—6 mm.

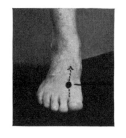

VIII.3 TRAE-TCHRONG
Hyperton:
    Phosphorus 30—M
Hypersed:
    Cuprum met 6—30
            (de la Fuÿe)
2—5 mm.

The bilateral Regulator points, hypertonifying and hypersedative, on each of the three Centripetal YIN meridians:

   IV.   Kidneys
  VIII.   Liver
  XII.   Spleen—Pancreas

Passage Points on meridians I. V. & IX.

I.

The Passage point connecting Meridians I (heart) and II (Small intestine) is at I.5

Anatomical position: Bilateral: above the most prominent edge of the inferior apophysis of ulna, proximal to the internal end of the wrist fold.

Polarity of Treatment: Sedative, needle 2 mm—6 mm. Action is taken at this point whenever the indications are that meridian I is YANG *and* meridian II is YIN.

Homœopathic remedy: PHOSPHORUS 6—30 (de la Fuÿe)

V.

The Passage point, connecting Meridians V (Circulation-Sexfield) and VI (Three-Heater) is at V.6

Anatomical position: Bilateral: on the centre line of the anterior aspect of the forearm, about 6 cm above the wrist-fold (one fifth of the line wrist-fold to elbow-fold).

Polarity of Treatment: Sedative, needle 3 mm—2 cm. Action is taken at this point whenever the indications are that meridian V is YANG *and* meridian VI is YIN.

Homœopathic remedy: CALCAREA CARB 30—200 (de la Fuÿe)

IX.

The Passage point connecting meridians IX (Lungs) and X (Large intestine) is at IX.7

Anatomical position: Bilateral: on the anterior aspect of the wrist, in the radial groove 2 cm above the lower extremity of the radius.

Polarity of Treatment: Sedative, needle 2 mm—1 cm. Action is taken at this point whenever the indications are that meridian IX is YANG *and* meridian X is YIN.

Homœopathic remedy: PHOSPHORUS 6 (de la Fuÿe)

46

PS

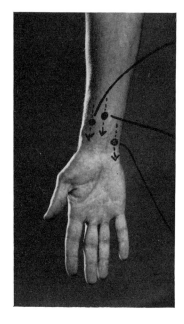

IX.7 LIE-TSIUE (PS to X)
Phosphorous 6
(de la Fuÿe)
2 mm—1 cm.

V.6 NEI-KOANN (PS to VI)
calcarea carb. 30—200
(de la Fuÿe)
3 mm—2 cm.

I.5 TRONG-LI (PS to II)
phosphorus 6—30
(de la Fuÿe)
2—6 mm.

The bilateral Passage points (PS) on each of the three Centrifugal YIN organ meridians:

I.   Heart

V.   Circulation-Sexfield

IX. Lungs

NOTE: *For a different orientation towards the correct use of passage points see note in Chapter on Treatment.*

Passage points on meridians II. VI. & X.

II.

The Passage point connecting meridian II (Small intestine) and I (Heart) is at II. 7

Anatomical position: Bilateral: on the postero-internal aspect of the forearm, at the mid-point of a line drawn between the wrist-fold and elbow-fold.

Polarity of Treatment: Sedative, needle 2 mm—6 mm.
Action is taken at this point whenever the indications are that meridian II is YANG *and* meridian I is YIN

Homœopathic remedy: VERAT ALB 6—30 (de la Fuÿe)

VI.

The Passage point connecting meridians VI (Three-Heater) and V (Circulation-Sexfield) is at VI.5

Anatomical position: Bilateral: on the posterior aspect of the forearm, 6 cm above the infero-external of the ulna apophysis (radial side of ulna).

Polarity of Treatment: Sedative, needle 5 mm—1 cm.
Action is taken at this point whenever the indications are that meridian VI is YANG *and* meridian V is YIN.

Homœopathic remedy: PHOSPHORUS 6 (de la Fuÿe)

X.

The Passage point connecting meridians X (Large intestine) and IX (Lungs) is at X.6

Anatomical position: Bilateral: on the external aspect of the forearm at the junction of the lower and middle third of a line drawn from the inferior extremity of the radial apophysis to the external of head of radius.

Polarity of Treatment: Sedative, needle 2 mm—1 cm.
Action is taken at the point whenever the indications are that meridian X is YANG *and* meridian IX is YIN.

Homœopathic remedy: ANTIMON TAR 6 (de la Fuÿe)

PS

Passage points

II, VI, X.

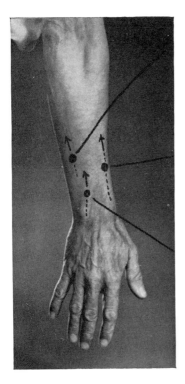

II.7 TCHE-TCHENG (PS to I)
verat. alb. 6—30
(de la Fuÿe)
2—6 mm.

X.6 PIENN-LI (PS to IX)
Antimon. tar. 6
(de la Fuÿe)
2 mm—1 cm.

VI.5 OAE-KOANN (PS to V)
phosphorus 6 (de la Fuÿe)
5 mm—1 cm.

The bilateral Passage points (PS) on each of the three Centripetal
YANG organ meridians:

    II.   Small Intestine

    VI.   Thermo-Regulator or Three-Heater

    X.   Large Intestine

NOTE: *For a different orientation towards the correct use of
passage points see note in Chapter on Treatment.*

Passage points on meridians III. VII. & XI.

III.

The Passage point connecting meridians III (Bladder) and IV (Kidneys) is at III.58

Anatomical position: Bilateral: on the postero-extern of the leg, half-way between the external malleolus and the tibio-femoral articulation, on the external gastrocnemius.

Polarity of Treatment: Sedative, needle 6 mm—2 cm.
Action is taken at this point whenever indications are that meridian III is YANG *and* meridian IV is YIN.

Homœopathic remedy: MEDORRHINUM 6—M (de la Füye)

VII.

The Passage point connecting meridians VII (Gall Bladder) and VIII (Liver) is at VII.37

Anatomical position: Bilateral: on the antero-external aspect of the leg, 6 cm below the middle of a line drawn from the anterior tuberosity of the tibial plateau to the external malleolus.

Polarity of Treatment: Sedative, needle 4 mm.
Action is taken at this point whenever the indications are that meridian VII is YANG and meridian VIII is YIN.

Homœopathic remedy: MYRICA 3—12 (de la Füye)

XI.

The Passage point connecting meridians XI (Stomach) and XII (Spleen-Pancreas) is at XI.40

Anatomical position: Bilateral: on the antero-extern of the leg, anterior edge of the fibula, 2 cm above the middle of a line drawn from the external malleolus to the anterior tuberosity of tibia.

Polarity of Treatment: Sedative, needle 2 mm—1 cm.
Action is taken at this point whenever the indications are that meridian XI is YANG *and* meridian XII is YIN.

Homœopathic remedy: MOSCHUS 3—6 (de la Füye)

PS

Passage points

III, VII, XI.

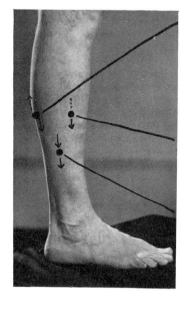

III.58 FEI-IANG (PS to IV)
medorrhinum 6—M
(de la Fuÿe)
6 mm—2 cm.

XI.40 FONG-LONG (PS to XII)
moschus 3—6
(de la Fuÿe)
2 mm—1 cm.

VII.37 KOANG-MING
(PS to VIII)
myrica 3—12
(de la Fuÿe)
4 mm.

The bilateral Passage points on each of the three Centrifugal YANG organ meridians:

III.   Bladder

VII.   Gall-Bladder

XI.   Stomach

NOTE: *For a different orientation towards the correct use of passage points see note in Chapter on Treatment.*

51

Passage points on meridians IV. VIII. & XII.

IV.

The Passage point connecting meridians IV (Kidneys) and III (Bladder) is at IV.4

Anatomical position: Bilateral: 1 cm behind the internal malleolus at the horizontal level of the most prominent part of the malleolus.

Polarity of Treatment: Sedative, needle 2 mm—6 mm.
Action at this point is taken whenever the indications are that meridian IV is YANG and meridian III is YIN.

Homœopathic remedy: EQUISETUM 1x—6 (de la Fuÿe)

VIII.

The Passage point connecting meridian VIII (Liver) and VII (Gall bladder) is at VIII.6

Anatomical position: Bilateral: on the antero-internal aspect of the leg on the centre line of the tibia, about 4 cm below the midpoint of a line drawn from the internal malleolus to the antero-intern of the tibio-femoral articulation.

Polarity of Treatment: Sedative, needle 2 mm—6 mm.
Action is taken at this point whenever the indications are that meridian VIII is YANG *and* meridian VII is YIN.

Homœopathic remedy: CHELIDONIUM 3x—6 (de la Fuÿe)

XII.

The Passage point connecting meridians XII (Spleen-Pancreas) and XI (Stomach) is at XII.4

Anatomical position: Bilateral: on the internal aspect of the foot, just below the articulation of the first metatarsal and the first cuniform (in the angle of these two bones).

Polarity of Treatment: Sedative, needle 2 mm—8 mm.
Action is taken at this point whenever the indications are that meridian XII is YANG *and* meridian XI is YIN.

Homœopathic remedies: PODOPHYLLUM 6—12 (de la Fuÿe)
SEPIA 6—12 (de la Fuÿe)

PS

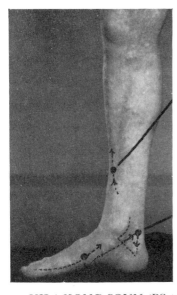

VIII.6 LI-KEOU (PS to VII)
  chelidonium 3x—6
    (de la Fuÿe)
  2—6 mm.

IV.4 TA-TCHONG (PS to III)
  equisetum 1x—6
    (de la Fuÿe)
  2—6 mm.

XII.4 KONG-SOUN (PS to XI)
  podophyllum 6—12 (right side)
    (de la Fuÿe)
  sepia 6—30 left side
    (de la Fuÿe)
  2—8 mm.

The bilateral Passage points on each of the three Centripetal YIN organ meridians:

  IV. Kidneys

  VIII. Liver

  XII. Spleen-Pancreas

NOTE: *For a different orientation towards the correct use of passage points see note in Chapter on Treatment.*

53

Vesical re-inforcement points of meridians I. V. & IX.

I.

The Vesical re-inforcement point of meridian I (Heart) is at III.15

Anatomical position: Bilateral: between the transverse processes of the fifth and sixth dorsal vertebrae.

Polarity of Treatment: Tonification or Sedative, needle 2 mm—2 cm.

Homœopathic remedies: GELSEMIUM 6 left side (Weihe)
KALI CARB 6 right side (de la Fuÿe)

V.

The Vesical re-inforcement point of meridian V (Circulation-Sexfield) is at III.14

Anatomical position: Bilateral: between the transverse processes of the fourth and fifth dorsal vertebrae.

Polarity of Treatment: Tonification or Sedative, needle 4 mm—2 cm.

Homœopathic remedy: AGARICUS 6—30 left side (de la Fuÿe)
right side (Weihe)

IX.

The Vesical re-inforcement point of meridian IX (Lungs) is at III.13

Anatomical position: Bilateral: between the transverse processes of the third and fourth dorsal vertebrae.

Polarity of Treatment: Tonification or Sedative
needle 2 mm—2 cm.

Homœopathic remedy: ANTIMON TAR 6—30 (de la Fuÿe)

VR

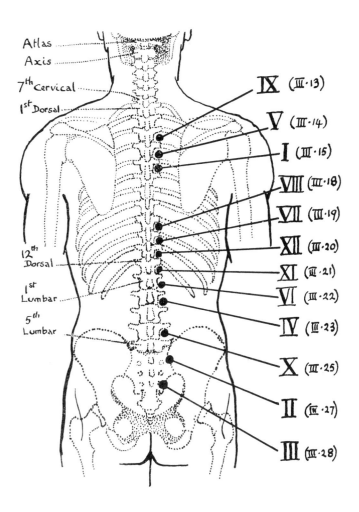

IX	(III·13)
V	(III·14)
I	(III·15)
VIII	(III·18)
VII	(III·19)
XII	(III·20)
XI	(III·21)
VI	(III·22)
IV	(III·23)
X	(III·25)
II	(IV·27)
III	(III·28)

Atlas
Axis
7th Cervical
1st Dorsal
12th Dorsal
1st Lumbar
5th Lumbar

*All these points are bilateral though, in this
diagram, one side only is marked*

55

Vesical re-inforcement points of meridians II. VI. & X.

II.

The Vesical re-inforcement point of meridian II (Small intestine) is at III.27

Anatomical position: Bilateral: on the postero-superior iliac spine, 4 cm lateral to the first sacral foramen.

Polarity of Treatment: Tonification or Sedative,
                              needle 2 mm—1 cm.

Homœopathic Remedy: CANTHARIS 6 (de la Fuÿe)

VI.

The Vesical re-inforcement point of meridian VI (Three Heater) is at III.22

Anatomical position: Bilateral: between the transverse processes of the first and second lumbar vertabrae.

Polarity of Treatment: Tonification or Sedative,
                              needle 2 mm—2 cm.

Homœopathic remedy: ARGENTUM NIT 6—30 (de la Fuÿe)

X.

The Vesical re-inforcement point of meridian X (Large intestine) is at III.25

Anatomical position: Bilateral: between the transvere processes of the fourth and fifth lumbar vertebrae.

Polarity of Treatment: Tonification or Sedative,
                              needle 2 mm—2 cm.

Homœopathic remedy: ALOE 6—30 (de la Fuÿe)

Vesical re-inforcement points of meridians III. VII. & XI.

III.

The Vesical re-inforcement point of meridian III (Bladder) is at III.28

Anatomical position: Bilateral: 6 cm from and slightly below the third sacral foramen. (Chamfrault places it at 4 cm lateral to the second sacral foramen).

Polarity of Treatment: Tonification or Sedative, needle 2 mm—1 cm.

Homœopathic remedy: PAREIRA BRAVA 3 (de la Fuÿe)

VII.

The Vesical re-inforcement point of meridian VII (Gall bladder) is at III.19

Anatomical position: Bilateral: between the transverse processes of the tenth and eleventh dorsal vertebrae.

Polarity of Treatment: Tonification or Sedative, needle 2 mm—2 cm.

Homœopathic remedy: BERBERIS 6 (de la Fuÿe)

XI.

The Vesical re-inforcement point of meridian XI (Stomach) is at III.21

Anatomical position: Bilateral: between the transverse processes of the twelfth dorsal and the first lumbar vertebrae.

Polarity of Treatment: Tonification or Sedative, needle 6 mm—2 cm.

Homœopathic remedies:
Tonification: ABROTANUM 3—6 (de la Fuÿe)
Sedative: AETHUSA 3—6 (de la Fuÿe)

Vesical re-inforcement points of meridians IV. VIII. & XII.

IV.

The Vesical re-inforcement point of meridian IV (Kidneys) is at III.23

Anatomical position: Bilateral: between the transverse processes of the second and third lumbar vertebrae (external extremities).

Polarity of Treatment: Tonification or Sedative, needle 6 mm—2 cm.

Homœopathic remedy: TEREBENTHINA 6—12 (de la Fuÿe)

VIII.   .

The Vesical re-inforcement point of meridian VIII (Liver) is at III.18

Anatomical position: Bilateral: between the transverse processes of the ninth and tenth dorsal vertebrae

Polarity of Treatment: Tonification or Sedative, needle 6 mm—2 cm.

Homœopathic remedy: FABIANA IMBRICATA TM—6 (de la Fuÿe)

XIII.

The Vesical re-inforcement point of meridian XII (Spleen-Pancreas) is at III.20

Anatomical position: Bilateral: between the transverse processes of the eleventh and twelfth dorsal vertebrae.

Polarity of Treatment: Tonification or Sedative, needle 2 mm—2 cm.

Homœopathic remedy: CEANOTHUS 6—30 (de la Fuÿe)

GOVERNOR & CONCEPTION VESSEL MERIDIANS

The points on the two median Vessel meridians, which are purely functional meridians and not specifically linked to any internal organs, are arranged as follows: —

PIII(i), the Governor Vessel Meridian, is considered in two sections. The first section, which concerns 'physical' energy, is from the tip of he coccyx to the seventh cervical vertebra (.13); the second section, which concerns 'psychic' energy, is from the seventh cervical vertebra (.13bis) to the last point on the gum between the two upper front teeth.

PIV(i), the Conception Vessel Meridian, is considered in three sections. The first section, dealing with the genito-urinary function, is from the perineum to the umbilicus. The second section, dealing with the digestive function, is from the umbilicus to the xiphoid process; and the third section, which concerns the respiratory function, is from the xiphoid process to the chin.

On these meridians there are no Toning nor Sedative points, each point being treated in tonification or in sedation according to the symptoms.

There are considerable discrepancies among the various authorities regarding the exact placing of many of the points on these two meridians. For the sake of consistency in this present work we have followed the placing and numbering as given by Dr. de la Fuÿe. This does not mean to say, however, that we have necessarily accepted these positions as the soundest and most authoritative, but rather that, for practical purposes, it is expedient to do so, especially in view of the extensive clinical experience of Dr. de la Fuÿe.

The flow of Vital Force in both of these meridians is continuous and vertically upwards. We have not yet read any satisfactory indication of how the circuit of each of these is completed: our own *tentative* view is that PIII(i) follows the anterior median line of the spine downwards; and that PIV(i) follows the path of the larynx, trachea, bronchi and, in a general way, the lungs, then the general line of the entire alimentary tract.

This we have represented diagramatically thus: —

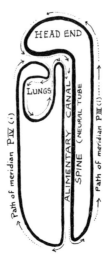

We are well aware that our reasons for holding this *tentative* view may appear nonsensical, and without scientific basis, to persons who discount "intuition" or who have no time for preposterous thinking. It is our belief that all the really significant advances ever made by Man, in cultural progress, have come about because somewhere along the line there have been people who have dared to think "preposterously".

We were not able to visualize a perpetual one-way stream of Vital Force, beginning at one point and finishing at another. We felt that some circuit there must be. We observed that, according to the traditional Chinese placing of the 'beginning' and 'ending' points of the meridians PIII(i) and PIV(i), these points appeared at either end of the alimentary canal; what, therefore, could be more natural than for the circuit to be continuous *through* this canal?

"Physical" man can be considered as a mobile tube, moving through environment in the general direction of the 'head end.' To us this extremely simplified conception appeared to agree with the Yang-Yin science classification of man as a YIN Being.*

> * see the chapter on Chinese Science (sections Biology and Medicine) in Sakurazawa's Principe Unique.

As in fact there is no break in the continuity of the skin, the regions where outside-the-skin-environment (gases, liquids, solids, etc.) becomes assimilated and transformed into an inside-the-skin-event would be of especial significance.

"Physical" environment becomes transformed into an inside-the-skin-event at two chief places (i) in the lungs, and (ii) in the intestines: and inside-the-skin becomes an outside-the-skin event wherever secretions from any gland or organ enter the alimentary tract and gases are liberated into the air.

Man's "Psychic" environment, though filtered through receptors of stimuli (eyes, ears, etc.) and converted into assimilable form, *somewhere becomes transformed into* an inside-the-skin or inside-the-brain happening.

We have elected to look upon, at least tentatively, the various nerve plexi, etc., as the "assimilating areas" comparable to the lungs and intestines.

With these notions we are able to look upon the two meridians PIII(i) and PIV(i) as means of controlling the operation of 'physical and psychic' environment becoming man, and man becoming environment 'physical and psychic'.

It needs also to be borne in mind that man *is not* a merely passive transformer of environmnet as are plants and animals, for it is a human characteristic that man is able to exercise positive and 'conscious' control and therefore must be looked upon as belonging to a *creative class of life*.

As we have already intimated, this may well be looked upon as speculation (even nonsensical) nevertheless, however unscientifically or inadequately we have expressed these notions, it may happen that one day these words will fecundate, and start a chain of thought somewhere in someone leading eventually to a worthwhile discovery and an adequately formulated theory.

61

Points on the Governor Vessel Meridian PIII (i) (Section I) from the tip of the coccyx to the seventh cervical vertebra.

.1 (not listed by de la Fuÿe)

Anatomical position: median; on the point of the coccyx.

Polarity of Treatment: Ton or Sed according to symptoms. needle .5 cm (Stiefvater)

.2 (not listed by de la Fuÿe)

Anatomical position: median; just above the sacro-coccygeal articulation.

Polarity of Treatment: Ton or Sed according to symptoms. needle 2 mm—4 mm (Stiefvater)

.3

Anatomical position: median on the point of the spinous process of the fifth lumbar vertebra.

Polarity of Treatment: Usually Sedative, needle 2 mm—5 mm.

Homœopathic remedy: HYPERICUM 3x—6 (Weihe)

.3bis (.3 according to Stiefvater)

Anatomical position: median; on the point of the spinous process of the fourth lumbar vertabra.

Polarity of Treatment: Ton or Sed, needle 4 mm—5 mm.

Homœopathic remedies:
In Tonification GINSENG TM-3x   (de la Fuÿe)
in Sedation, male STAPHYSAGRIA 200 (de la Fuÿe)
            female MUREX 30   (de la Fuÿe)
            female ORIGANUM 6   (de la Fuÿe)
            URANIUM NITRICUM 6—200 (Weihe)

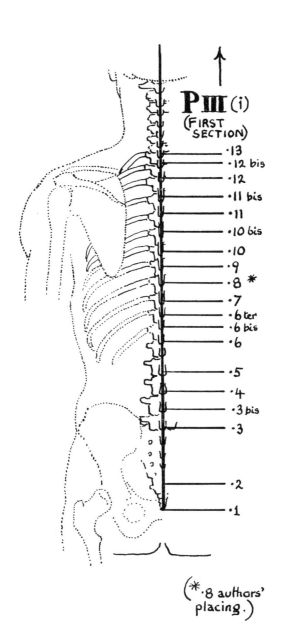

P III (i)

(FIRST SECTION)

· 13
· 12 bis
· 12
· 11 bis
· 11
· 10 bis
· 10
· 9
· 8   *
· 7
· 6 ter
· 6 bis
· 6
· 5
· 4
· 3 bis
· 3

· 2

· 1

$\left(\substack{* \\ \cdot 8} \text{ authors'} \atop \text{placing.} \right)$

63

.4

    Anatomical position: median; on the spinous process of the third lumbar vertebra (2nd l.v. according to Stiefvater)

    Polarity of Treatment: usually Tonification, needle 5 mm.

    Homœopathic remedy: SELENIUM 30—M (Weihe)

.5

    Anatomical position: median; on the spinous process of the second lumbar vertebra (1st l.v. according to Stiefvater)

    Polarity of Treatment: Usually Sedative, needle 2—5 mm.

    Homœopathic remedy: ARGENTUM NITRICUM 6 — 12 (Weihe)

.6

    Anatomical position: median; on the spinous process of the twelfth dorsal vertebra (10th d.v. according to Stiefvater)

    Polarity of Treatment: usually Sedative, needle 2 mm—5 mm.

    Homœopathic remedy: CORALLIUM RUBRUM 30—200 (Weihe)

.6bis   (not listed by Stiefvater)

    Anatomical position: median; on spinous process of the eleventh dorsal vertebra.

    Polarity of Treatment: usually Tonification, needle 2—4 mm.

    Homœopathic remedy: BUFO 30—200 (Weihe)

.6ter (not listed by de la Fuÿe, .6 according to Stiefvater)

Anatomical position: median; on the spinous process of the
10th dorsal vertebra.
Polarity of Treatment: Ton or Sed, needle .5 cm.

.7 (not listed by de la Fuÿe)

Anatomical position: median; on the spinous process of the
9th dorsal vertebra.
Polarity of Treatment: Ton or Sed, needle .5 cm.

.8 (not listed by de la Fuÿe, not at this position by Stiefvater)

Anatomical position: median; on the spinous process of the
eighth dorsal vertebra.

.9 (not listed by de la Fuÿe, .8 according to Stiefvater)

Anatomical position: median; on the spinous process of the
seventh dorsal vertebra.
Polarity of Treatment: Ton or Sed, needle .5 cm.

.10 (.9 according to Stiefvater)

Anatomical position: median; on the spinous process of the
sixth dorsal vertebra.
Polarity of Treatment: usually Tonification, needle 2—5 mm.
Homœopathic remedy: OSMIUM 30—200 (Weihe)

.10 bis (.10 according to Stiefvater)

Anatomical position: median; on the spinous process of the
fifth dorsal vertebra.
Polarity of Treatment: usually Tonification, needle 2—6 mm
Homœopathic remedy: TELLURIUM 200—M (Weihe)

.11

    Anatomical position: median; on the spinous process of the fourth dorsal vertebra.

    Polarity of Treatment: usually Sedative, needle 2 mm—8 mm.

    Homœopathic remedies:
              HYDROPHOBINUM 30—200 de la Fuÿe)
              STRAMONIUM 30—200 de la Fuÿe)

.11 bis (.11 according to Stiefvater)

    Anatomical position: median; on the spinous process of the third dorsal vertebra

    Polarity of Treatment: usually Sedative, needle 2—6 mm.

    Homœopathic remedy: PARIS QUADRIFOLIA 30 (Weihe)

.12

    Anatomical position: median; on the spinous process of the second dorsal vertebra.

    Polarity of Treatment: usually Sedative, needle 2 mm—5 mm.

    Homœopathic Remedy: COCA 6 (Weihe)

.12 bis (not listed by de la Fuÿe)
    Anatomical position: median; on the spinous process of the first dorsal vertebra.

    Polarity of Treatment: Ton or Sed, needle .5 mm.

.13

    Anatomical position: median; on the spinous process of the seventh cervical vertebra.

    Polarity of Treatment: Ton or Sed, needle 2—5 mm.

    Homœopathic remedy: PICRICUM ACIDUM 6—30 (Weihe)

P III (i)

.13   bis

Anatomical position: median, on the spinous process of the seventh cervical vertebra.

Polarity of Treatment: usually Tonification, needle 2 mm—5 mm.

Homœopathic remedy: CARBONEUM SULFURATUM 30
(Weihe)

.13   ter

Anatomical position: median, on the spinous process of the fourth cervical vertebra.

Polarity of Treatment: usually in Tonification, needle 4 mm.

Homœopathic remedy: LATHYRUS SATIVUS 30 (Weihe)

.14

Anatomical position: median, on the spinous process of the third cervical vertebra.

Polarity of Treatment: Ton or Sed, needle 4 mm.

Homœopathic remedy: MENYANTHES 6—30 (Weihe)

.15

Anatomical position: median, on the spinous process of the second cervical vertebra.

Polarity of Treatment: usually Sedative, needle 2 mm— 5mm.

Homœopathic remedy: CUPRUM ARSENICUM 3—6
(Weihe)

67

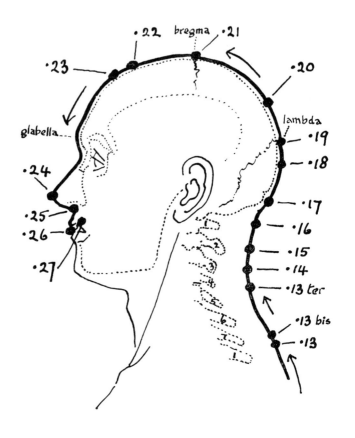

•22   bregma   •21

•23

•20

glabella

lambda

•19

•18

•24

•17

•25   •16

•26   •15

•27   •14

•13 ter

•13 bis

•13

68

.16

Anatomical position: median, postero-inferior occiput, at the level of the atlanto-occipital articulation.

Polarity of Treatment: usually Sedative, needle 2 mm—5 mm.

Homœopathic remedy: RHUS RADICANS 6 (Weihe)

.17 (not listed by de la Füÿe)

Anatomical position: median, on the upper border of the occipital foramen.

Polarity of Treatment: Ton or Sed, needle 2 mm.

.18 (not listed by de la Füÿe)

Anatomical position: median, on the external occiptal protuberance.

Polarity of Treatment: Ton or Sed, needle 2 mm.

.19

Anatomical position: median, at the parieto-occipital suture (lambda).

Polarity of Treatment: Ton or Sed. needle 2 mm.

Homœopathic remedy:
in Tonification: ZINCUM MET 30—200(de la Füÿe)
in Sedation: THERIDION .30—200 (de la Füÿe)

.20 (not listed by de la Füÿe)

Anatomical postion: median, half-way between lambda and bregma; about 6 cm above parieto-occipital suture.

Polarity of Treatment: Ton or Sed. needle 2 mm.

69

.21　(not listed by de la Fuÿe)
Anatomical position: median, at the meeting of the saggital suture and frontal bone.
Polarity of Treatment: Ton or Sed, needle 2 mm.

.22　(not listed by de la Fuÿe)
Anatomical position: median, on the frontal bone 3 cm from .21
Polarity of Treatment: Ton or Sed, 2 mm.

.23　(not listed by de la Fuÿe)
Anatomical position: median on the frontal bone, halfway between bregma and glabella.
Polarity of Treatment: Ton or Sed, needle 2 mm.

.24　(not listed by de la Fuÿe)
Anatomical position: on the tip of the nose.
Polarity of Treatment: Ton or Sed, needle 2 mm.

.25　(not listed by de la Fuÿe)
Anatomical position: median, on the orbicularis oris, just under the anterior nasal spine.
Polarity of Treatment: Ton or Sed, needle 2 mm.

.26　(not listed by de la Fuÿe, listed by Stitfvater as "not used".)
Anatomical position: median, on the upper lip, below the lower extremeity of the naso-labial fold.
Polarity of Treatment: probably Sedative (see Appendix B) needle 1 mm.

.27　(not listed by de la Fuÿe)
Anatomical position: median, inside the mouth, on the front of the gum just above the first incisors of the upper jaw.
Polarity of Treatment: Ton or Sed, needle 1 mm. (Stiefvater).

SECTION I.

.1   (not listed by de la Fuÿe)

Anatomical position: Median, halfway between the scrotum or vulva and the anus.

Polarity of Treatment: probably Sedative, needle 1 cm.
(Stiefvater)

.2

Anatomical Position: Median, on the superior border of the pubis symphysis.

Polarity of Treatment: usually Sedative, needle 3 mm—1 cm.

Homœopathic remedy: FERRUM IODATUM 3x (Weihe)

.3

Anatomical Position: Median 4 cm above the pubis symphysis

Polarity of Treatment: usually Sedative, needle 2 mm—2 cm.

Homœopathic remedy: RHUS TOX 3—12 (Weihe)

.4

Anatomical Position: Median, at the junction of the lower and middle third of a line drawn from the umbilicus to the upper border of the pubis symphysis.

Polarity of Treatment: Ton or Sed, needle 5 mm—2 cm.

Homœopathic remedy: HYDRASTIS 6—30 (Weihe)

71

.5

Anatomical Position: Median, at the junction of the upper and middle quarter of a line drawn from the umbilicus to the lower border of the pubis symphysis.

Polarity of Treatment: usually Sedative, needle 5 mm—2 cm.

Homœopathic remedy: PHOSPHORUS 6—30 (de la Fuÿe)

.6

Anatomical Position: Median, 4 cm below the umbilicus.

Polarity of Treatment: usually Ton. needle 5 mm—2 cm.

Homœopathic remedy: SILICEA 200—M (de la Fuÿe)

.7

Anatomical Position: Median, 2 cm below the umbilicus.

Polarity of Treatment: usually Sed., needle 4 mm—2 cm.

Homœopathic remedy: CANTHARIS 6—200 (de la Fuÿe)

SECTION II

.8   (not listed by de la Fuÿe)

Anatomical position: Median, on the umbilicus.
Polarity of Treatment: Ton or Sed. needle 5 mm—1 cm.
                                                    (Stiefvater)
N.B. Traditionally forbidden to needle. Use moxa after
having filled the umbilicus with salt.

.9

Anatomical Position: Median, 2 cm. above umbilicus.
Polarity of Treatment: usually Sedative, needle 4 mm—2 cm.
Homœopathic remedy: SILICEA 30—200 (Weihe).

.10   (not listed by de la Fuÿe)

Anatomical position: Median, 5 cm above the umbilicus.
Polarity of Treatment: Ton or Sed., needle 5 mm—2 cm.
                                                    (Stiefvater).

.11

Anatomical position: Median, 2 cm. below the centre of a
                     line drawn from the umbilicus to the
                     superior part of the xiphoid process.
Polarity of Treatment: usually Sedative, needle 6 mm—2 cm.
Homœopathic remedy: MEZERUM 30 (Weihe)

.11 bis

Anatomical position: Median, exactly halfway between the
                     umbilicus and the superior part of the
                     xiphoid process.
Polarity of Treatment: Ton or Sed. needle 6 mm.
Homœopathic remedy: IODIUM 6, 30, 200 (Weihe)

73

.12

Anatomical position: Median, 2 cm. above the centre of the line drawn from the umbilicus to the superior part of the xiphoid process, at the level of the sterno-costal angles.

Polarity of Treatment: usually Sedative, needle 6 mm.

.13

Anatomical position: Median, $\frac{3}{8}$ths of the distance between xiphoid process and umbilicus.

Polarity of Treatment: usually Sedative, needle 10—16mm.

Homœopathic remedy: CUPRUM MET 6—30 (de la Fuÿe)

.14

Anatomical position: Median, $\frac{1}{8}$th of the distance from the xiphoid process to umbilicus, solar plexus.

Polarity of Treatment: usually sedative needle 4 mm—1 cm.

Homœopathic remedy: TABACUM 12—30 (de la Fuÿe)
IPECA 6—12 (Weihe)

.14 bis

Anatomical position: Median, just less than 2 cm. below the tip of the xiphoid process.

Polarity of Treatment: usually Sedative, needle 3 mm.

Homœopathic remedy: VERAT ALB 3—6 (Weihe)

74

SECTION III   (Conception Vessel)

.15

    Anatomical position: Median, just below the tip of the
                            xiphoid process.
    Polarity of Treatment: Ton or Sed needle 5 mm—1 cm.
    Homœopathic remedy: PHOSPHORIC ACID 3, 6, 30
                                                (de la Fuÿe)

.16

    Anatomical position: Median, on the superior base of the
                            xiphoid.
    Polarity of Treatment: usually Sedative, needle 1 mm—4 mm.
    Homœopathic remedy: PHOSPHORUS 6—30 (de la Fuÿe)

.16   bis

    Anatomical position: Median, on the sternum at the level of
                            the fifth intercostal space.
    Polarity of Treatment: usually Ton. needle 4 mm.
    Homœopathic remedy: ARGENTUM MET 6 (Weihe)

.17

    Anatomical position: Median, on the sternum at the level of
                            the fourth intercostal space.
    Polarity of Treatment: usually Sedative, needle 1 mm—4 mm.
    Homœopathic remedy: RAPHANUS SATIVUS 6 (Weihe)

.18

    Anatomical position: Median, on the sternum at the level of
                            the third intercostal space.
    Polarity of Treatment: usually Sedative, needle 1 mm—4 mm.
    Homœopathic remedy: MERCURIUS IODATUS RUBER 6
                                                (Weihe)

.19

    Anatomical position: Median, on the sternum at the level of the second intercostal space.

    Polarity of Treatment: usually Sedative, needle 1 mm—4 mm.

    Homœopathic remedy: CALCAREA IODATA 6 (Weihe)

.20

    Anatomical position: Median, on the sternum at the level of the first intercostal space.

    Polarity of Treatment: usually Sedative, needle 1 mm—4 mm.

    Homœopathic remedy: BROMIUM 3—6 (Weihe)

.21 & .22

    Anatomical positions:

        .21 median, on the sternum between the clavicle and first rib.

        .22 median 2 cm above the superior border of the manubrium.

    Polarity of Treatment: usually Sedative, needles 1—5 mm.

    Homœopathic remedy: RUMEX CRISPUS 3—6 (Weihe)

.23 (not listed by de la Fuÿe)

    Anatomical position: Median, in the angle between the throat and underneath part of the chin.

    Polarity of Treatment: needle 1 mm—5 mm. (Stiefvater)

.24 (not listed by de la Fuÿe)

    Anatomical position: median, between the lower lip and the point of the chin.

    Polarity of Treatment: needle 1 mm—2 mm (Stiefvater)

.25 (not included in traditional Acupuncture points)

    Anatomical position: median, on the lower lip where it touches the upper lip.

    Polarity of Treatment: probably Sedative(see Appendix B) needle 1 mm.

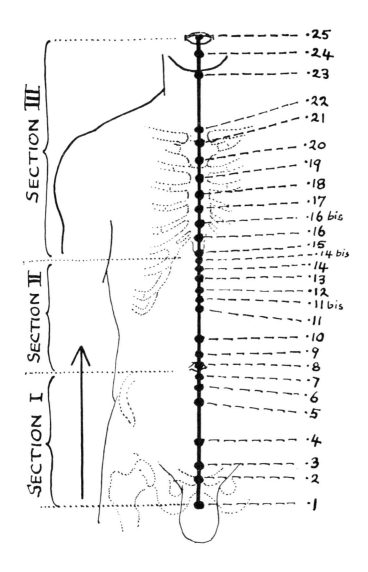

SECTION III

SECTION II

SECTION I

•25
•24
•23
•22
•21
•20
•19
•18
•17
•16 bis
•16
•15
•14 bis
•14
•13
•12
•11 bis
•11
•10
•9
•8
•7
•6
•5
•4
•3
•2
•1

TREATMENT METHODS

In this handbook we concern ourselves with three methods of treatment only: Massage, Moxa, and Needles. These are given in order of simplicity. There are other methods involving the use of high frequency electricity, diathermy, ultra-sonics, and so on. These have been briefly mentioned in our Chinese System of Healing.

MASSAGE: the simplest of all methods, requiring no instruments nor equipment of any kind. This method is without doubt as effective as any other, and, in many instances, is preferable especially when treating the very young, very old, or nervous patients.

Massage in Tonification

This is given with the point of one finger, or with the fingernail, in a sort of boring circulatory movement. The finger (or fingernail) must *not* move over the skin: the skin and underlying tissues should move as one with the finger, as in the Swedish deep friction movement.

If the points are bilateral, both sides must be treated simultaneously.

When the treatment has been continued for long enough the practitioner will detect a *'change of feel' in* the texture of the area massaged. We do not know of a really suitable verbal description of this 'change of feel', but once this has been experienced it will instantly be recognized again.

At any one treatment one never massages in Tonification *and* in Sedation on the same meridian; either one *or* the other, never both.

Massage in Sedation

This takes the form of a light stroking movement with the tips of one or two fingers (a *very light* effleurage) *in the direction of the flow of Tsri*. The direction of this flow at each point is clearly indicated in the diagrams.

If the points are bilateral, both sides must be treated simultaneously.

When the treatment has been given for long enough the practitioner will detect a subtle change which might be described as there no longer being any 'drag'. One soon learns to recognize this change of feel.

MOXA

Modern practitioners (in the West) use what is known as a Moxa Hammer (see photo illustration). The head of the hammer is heated over a spirit flame for a few seconds.

Tonification: the pointed end of the hammer head is held on the point to be treated, and applied with some pressure.

Sedation: the rounded surface of the hammer head is lightly applied for Sedative effect.

The traditional, and without doubt the most effective, way is by burning a small cone of artemesia at the point selected. The herb itself seems to have curative properties.

NEEDLES

In Tonification. For this purpose specially made gold needles are inserted to the indicated depth. They are left in position until, in response to a gentle pull, the flesh *lets them be removed easily.* This may be after they have been in for any time up to fifteen or twenty minutes. Bilateral points must be treated simultaneously.

In Sedation. For this purpose specially made silver needles are inserted to the indicated depth, and left in position until the flesh lets them be removed easily.

Note: Some practitioners prefer to use steel needles, which are suitable for either Tonification or Sedative action. Fine steel needles with haft of copper wire (wound around the steel shaft) are the *traditional* needles.

79

Note on treatment at Passage Points.

There are two diametrically opposed doctrines as to the direction of flow of energy through the passages or channels linking the paired organ-meridians; and consequently the polarity of treatment to be given at the Passage Points also differs. To obviate confusion it appears essential that we make some attempt to clarify the position.

In this *book* we have taken Dr. Roger de la Fuÿe, a leading authority in France, as representative of Western Acupuncture based upon Soulié de Morant and practised in Hospitals and Clinics all over Europe. *Clinical results have shewn this westernized adaptation of oriental acupuncture to be therapeutically valid.*

On the other hand the Pure Chinese Tradition, as represented by Dr. Wu Wei Ping, gives an exactly opposite teaching in relation to Passage Points, as well as disagreeing in other respects. But, let us remember, the *Pure Chinese Tradition has proved itself therapeutically valid over many, many centuries.*

Dr. de la Fuÿe teaches that: If one meridian shows an Excess and the meridian with which it is paired shows a Deficiency, the balance is restored by acting in sedation upon the meridian having Excess.

Chinese Tradition "Purists", on the other hand, teach that: If a meridian shows an excess and the meridian with which it is paired shows a deficiency, the balance is restored by acting upon the deficient meridian in tonification.

De la Fuÿe seems to consider that *an excess accumulates because of impeded outflow* and therefore he indicates that dispersion action should be taken to remove the obstruction or reduce the activity of the restricting factor. The "Purists" teach that a *deficiency arises out of inadequate inflow* indicating a weakness of "suction" activity; therefore inflow needs stimulation at its point of entry.

Here then we have our two contradictory rules: (i) Sedate at the Passage point located on the meridian having Excess; (ii) Tonify at the Passage point located on the meridian having Deficiency.

Both schools recognize only ONE passage point on each meridian; both schools agree as to its location; and both maintain that energy can flow, in one direction only, through a Passage point. The contradiction reduces itself to a disagreement over the direction of flow. One says IN—the other says OUT!

In practice both achieve quite amazing therapeutic results.

A great part of our research work is devoted to looking for a resolution of just such apparent absurdities—*both are right.*

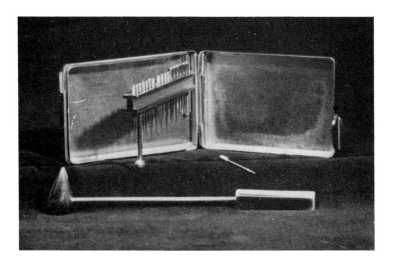

Authors' personal case of gold, silver and steel needles and a moxa hammer.

ALPHABETICAL REPERTORY

This repertory can be used in conjunction with the two repertories from Chinese System of Healing.

Abbreviations:

(TN) — Toning Point

(SD) — Sedative Point

(RG) — Regulator Point

(AL) — Alarm Point

(VR) — Vesical Re-inforcement Point

(PS to x) — Passage point to the meridian number which follows in Roman Numbers.

ton — action in tonification

sed — action in sedation

Note: Points listed are not necessarily given in order of importance. Selections and combinations will be a matter of individual evaluation according to the total picture of the patient.

REPERTORY

ABCESS
bones XII.5 (SD) sed.
dental abscess XII.5 (SD) sed., P IV (i) .9 sed.
fistula of lachrymal canal XII.5 (SD) sed., P IV (i) .9 sed.
throat I.5 (PS—II) sed., P IV (i) .21 & .22 sed.

ABDOMEN
cramp and distension of stomach P IV (i) .9 sed.
hard, painful, distended, inflated P IV (i) .9 sed.
hard and stretched P IV (i) .11 sed.
inflated P IV (i) .6 ton.
spasmodic pain in, see COLIC
tympanism with pains, especially during pregnancy
$\qquad$ P IV (i) .14 sed.

ABORTION
XII.4 (PS—XI) sed.

ACETONAEMIA
VIII.9 (TN) ton.

ACNE
IV.2 (SD) sed.

ADENITIS
V.7 (SD) sed., VIII.3 (RG) sed.

AEROCOLY
P IV (i) .17 (AI VI) sed.

AEROGASTRIA
III.15 (VR I) sed.,
P IV (i).17 (AL VI) sed. *or* P IV (i).6 ton.

84

AEROPHAGY
P IV (i) .17 (AL VI) sed.

AIR or GAS, distending tissue, see EMPHYSEMA
in colon P IV (i).17 sed.
in stomach P IV (i) .17 sed and III.15 (VRI) sed.
swallowing P IV (i).17 sed.

ALBUMINURIA
IV.II (AL V) sed.
III.65 (SD) sed.
III.64 (RG) sed.
I.5 (PS—II) sed.

ALCOHOLISM
XI.45 (SD) sed.
chronic P IV (i).6 ton.

AMENORRHOEA
XI.25 (AL.X) sed.
X.11 (TN) ton.
IV.2 (SD) sed.
VI.4 (RG) sed. or ton.

AMNESIA
I.9 (TN) ton.
IX.7 (PS—X) sed.
P III (i) .10 ton.
P III (i) .19 ton.

ANAEMIA
III.15 (VR I) ton.
III.67 (TN) ton.
VII.43 (TN) ton. or VII.24 (AL.VII) sed.
XII.15 (AL.XII) sed. and XII.5 (SD) sed.
or XII.2 (TN) ton. and XII.3 (RG) ton.
VI.3 (TN) ton.
P IV (i) .6 ton, P III (i) .4 ton.
special coupling Psychism Points
III.39 sed and XI.36 ton.

ANEURISM

IV.2 (SD) sed.

V.7 (RG) sed *or* V.9 (TN) ton.

V.7 (RG) ton.

ANGINA

I.9 (TN) ton. *or* I.7 (SD) sed.

P IV (i).14 (AL. I) sed.

V.1 (AL. V) sed.

V.7 (SD) sed. & III.14 (VR.V) sed.

IX.I (AL. IX) sed.

VI.3 (TN) ton, VI.4 (RG) ton. & III.22 (VR VI) sed.

XI.41 (TN) ton.

IV.3 (RG) sed.

ANGIOCHOLECYSTISIS

VII.25 (AL.IV) sed.

.24 (AL.VII) sed.

.23 (AL.VII) sed.

.38 (SD) sed. *or* .43 (TN) ton.

.40 (RG) sed. *or* .40 (RG) ton.

III.67 (TN) ton.

VIII.2 (SD) sed *or* VIII.9 (TN) ton.

VIII.6 (PS—VII) sed *or* VIII.3 (RG) ton.

ANOREXIA

XII.15 (AL XII) sed. *or* XII.3 (RG) ton.

III.64 (RG) ton.

VII.43 (TN) ton.

ANURIA

VIII.9 (TN) ton.

ANXIETY

P III (i).13 bis ton.

.19 ton.

(see Appendix B, 'e' zones and treatment of sympatheticotonia)

AORTITIS

I.7 (SD & RG) sed.

V.9 (TN) ton.

APATHY
    IV.7 (TN) ton.

APHASIA
    II.3 (TN) ton.

APOPLEXY
    P III (i).16 sed.   I.5 (PS—II) ton.

APPENDICITIS acute
    Special Point not on the meridians: Between the tibialis anticus and soleus, about two inches below the head of fibula. Sedative action.

    chronic VIII.2 & .3 (SD)
    P IV (i).6 ton.

APPETITE
    all disturbances of I.7 (SD) sed.
    none or excessive P IV (i).3 sed.
    lack of III.15 (VR.I) ton.
    XI.42 (RG) ton.

APPETITE, absence of, see ANOREXIA

ARTERIAL TENSION
        to raise   VIII.5 ton*
        to lower VIII.5 sed*

    * point known as the Bloodmaster,
      see Chinese System of Healing.

ARTERIOSCLEROSIS
    XII.15 (AL.XII) sed.
    I.7 (SD) sed.
    I.5 (PS—II) sed.
    III.15 (VR I) sed.
    IV.2 (SD) sed.
    IV.3 (RG) sed.

ARTERY WALLS, bulge in, see ANEURYSM

ARTHRITIS
    IV.2 (SD) sed.   VIII.2 (SD) sed.

87

ARYTHMY

    I.7 (SD) sed.

ASCITES

    P IV (i) .7 sed.
    XI.42 (RG) ton.

ASTHENIA

    P IV (i) .3 sed.

ASTHMA

    P IV (i) .5 (AL VI) sed.
           .17 (AL VI) sed.
      or .6 ton.
    VI.3 (TN) ton.
    VI.4 (RG) ton.
    IX.1 (AL IX) sed or if with emphysemia IX.9 (TN) ton.
    III.13 (VR IX) ton.
    III.67 (TN) ton.
    IV.3 (RG) sed.
    XII.15 (AL XII) sed.
    VIII.14 (AL VIII) sed. & VIII.2 (SD) sed.
    XI.40 (PS—XII) sed.

ATAXY

    II.4 (RG) ton.
    VI.3 (TN) ton.
    X.11 (TN) ton.
    locomotor add II.3 (TN) ton.

ATHREPSIA

    XI.42 (RG) ton.
    III.21 (VR XI) ton.
    VI.4 (RG) ton.
    P IV (i) .9 sed. *or* .6 ton.

ATONY

    all chronic states of II.4 (RG) ton.
    duodenal I.5 (PS-11) sed.
    large intestine X.4 (RG) ton.
    small intestine II.3 (TN) ton.

ATROPHY,
>progressive muscular II.3 (TN) ton.

AZOTAEMIA
>XI.25 (AL X) sed.

BACKWARDNESS, mental
>XII.2 (TN) ton.
>P III (i).6 bis ton.

BLADDER, inflammation of. see CYSTITIS

BLEEDING see HAEMORRHAGE
>from uterus, not connected with menstruation,
>>see METRORRHAGIA

BLENNORRHAGIA, BLENNORRHOEA
>III.65 (SD) sed.   )
>>.28 (VR III) sed.   )
>>.27 (VR II) sed.   )   or III.64 (RG) ton.
>>.22 (VR VI) sed.   )
>>.58 (PS-IV)   sed.   )
>P IV (i).7 sed.
>P IV (i).2 sed.

BLEPHARITIS
>X.4 (RG) ton.
>chronic, add XI.41 (TN) ton.

BLEPHARO-CONJUNCTIVITIS
>VII.37 (PS-VIII) sed.

BLOOD
>acetone in VIII.9 (TN) ton.
>deficiency of red corpuscles and/or haemoglobin
>>see ANAEMIA
>introgenous waste in (urea, etc.) XI.25 (AL X) sed.
>spitting   see HAEMOPTYSIS
>in urine, see HAEMATURIA
>vomiting, see HEAMATEMESIS

BOILS see FURONCULUS

BONES FEEL COLD IV.7 (TN) ton.

BRADYCARDIA
        I.9 (TN) ton.
        IV.7 (TN) ton.
        XII.3 (RG) ton *or* XII.4 (PS-XI) sed.

BREATH, bad V.7 (SD) sed.
        shortness of, see DYSPNOEA

BRIGHT'S DISEASE
        I.5 (PS-II) sed.
        IV.3 (RG) sed.
        III.23 (VR IV) sed.

BRONCHITIS
        P IV (i) .5 (AL VI) sed.
        IX.1 (AL IX) sed.
        IX.5 (SD) sed.
        IX.9 (RG & TN) ton *or* sed.
        IV.2 (SD) sed.
        VI.3 (TN) ton.
        VIII.2 (SD) sed.
        III.67 (TN) ton.
        V.9 (TN) ton.
        I.7 (RG) sed.
        III.14 (VR VI) sed.
        chronic P IV (i) .6 ton.
        III.13 (VR IX) ton.

BRONCHO-PNEUMONIA
        P IV (i).5 (AL VI) sed.
        IX.5 (SD) sed.
        VI.5 (PS-V) sed. *or* IX.7 (PS-X) sed.
        III.13 (VR IX) ton.
        IV.2 (SD) sed. and IV.3 (RG) sed.
        V.9 (TN) ton.

BULIMIA
    XII.15 (AL XII) sed.
    VII.40 (RG) ton.
    VI.4 (RG) sed.

CANCER
    XII.5 (SD) sed.
    VIII.3 (RG) sed.

    stomach
    XI.42 (RG) sed.
    III.23 (VR IV) sed.
    P IV (i) .12 (AL VI & XI) sed.
    XI.25 (AL X) sed.

CARDIAC DISORDERS,
    chronic P IV (i) .14 sed.

CATARACT
    VI.3 (TN) ton *or* VI.10 (SD) sed.
    III.64 (RG) ton.
    VIII.3 (RG) ton.

CHILDBIRTH,
    painful VI.5 (PS-V) sed.

CHILLINESS
    P IV (i) .9 sed.
    feeling of intense P IV (i) .6 ton.

CHOLECYSTITIS
    VII.23 (AL VII) sed.   )
    VII.24 (AL VII) sed.   )
    VII.38 (SD)   ) *or* VII.43 (TN) ton.
    VII.37 (PS-VIII) sed.   )   VII.40 (RG) ton.

    XII.15 (AL XII) sed.
    VIII.9 (TN) ton.
    VIII.3 (RG) ton.
    III.67 (TN) ton.
    IV.3 (RG) sed.

CHOLERA

> II.8 (SD) sed.
> .4 (RG) sed.
> .3 (TN) sed.
> IV.3 (RG) ton.
> infantile (severe form of infantile gastro-enteritis)
> III.21 (VR XI) sed.
> XII.4 (PS-XI) sed.

CHOLERIFORM

> affections II.7 (PS-I) sed.

CHOREA

> II.8 (SD) sed.
> IX.5 (SD) sed.
> III.14 (VR V) sed.

CIRRHOSIS

> XII.15 (AL XII) sed.
> VIII.9 (TN) ton.
> VIII.3 (RG) ton.
> VII.40 (RG) ton.
> IV.3 (RG) sed.

COLD

> icy feeling in hands and feet P III (i) .14 ton.
> intense feeling of (to the bones) PIII (i) .4 ton.
> IV.7 (TN) ton.
> common, see CORYZA

COLIC and diarrhoea with flatulence

> P IV (i) .3 sed.
>
> hepatic
> I.5 (PS-II) sed.
> IV.3 (RG) sed.
> V.6 (PS-VI) sed.
> VII.23 (AL VII) sed.
> VII.25 (AL IV) sed.
> VII.38 (SD) sed.
> VII.40 (RG) ton or sed.
> VII.43 (TN) ton.
> VIII.6 (PS-VII) sed.

VIII.3 (RG) ton or sed.
VIII.9 (TN) ton.
XII.15 (AL XII) sed.

hepatic and nephritic
III.23 (VR IV) sed.

intestinal
II.3 (TN) ton. or sed.
II.4 (RG) ton. or sed.

nephretic
III.28 (VR III) sed.
IV.4 (PS-III) sed.
VIII.25 (AL IV) sed.
VIII.9 (TN) ton.

COMA P III (i) .19 sed.

COMMON COLD, see CORYZA

CONGESTION,
cerebral
I.7 (RG & SD) sed.
III.64 (RG) sed.
VIII.2 (SD) sed.

liver
P IV (i) .2 sed.
XI.45 (SD) sed.
XII.15 (AL XII) sed.

portal
III.25 (VR X) sed.
XII.3 (RG) sed.

pulmonary
P IV (i) .5 (AL VI) sed.
III.13 (VR IX) ton.
IV.2 (SD) & .3 (RG) sed.
VI.4 (RG) sed.
VII.43 (TN) ton.
IX.5 (SD) sed.
    .7 (PS-X) sed.
    .9 (RG) sed.

CONJUNCTIVITIS

V.7 (SD) sed.
VI.5 (PS-V) sed.
X.4 (RG) ton.
XI.41 (TN) ton.
neonatorum X.2 & .3 (SD) sed.

CONSTIPATION

II.3 (TN) ton or (if chronic) II.7 (PS-I) sed.
II.4 (RG) ton.
III.25 (VR X) sed.
IV.1 (SD) sed or IV.3 (RG) ton.
VI.3 (TN) ton. or VI.4 (RG) sed.
VIII.2 (SD) sed. or VIII.9 (TN) ton.
XI.41 (TN) ton or (if chronic) XI.42 (RG) sed.
X.4 (RG) ton.
X.11 (TN) ton.
XI.25 (AL X) sed.
XII.5 (SD) sed.   XII.3 (RG) sed.
XII.15 (AL XII) sed.
P IV (i) .6 ton.

CONVULSIONS,

II.3 (TN) .4 (RG) & .8 (SD) sed.
III.14 (VR V) sed.
IX.5 (SD) sed.
XII.5 (SD) sed.
P III (i) .11 sed.
for all convulsions P IV (i) .15 ton or sed.

CORYZA

I.7 (SD & RG) sed.
III.64 (RG) sed *or* (if dry) ton.
X.4 (RG) ton.
XI.45 (SD) sed.

chronic
P III (i) .19 ton.
P IV (i) .4 sed.

COUGH

catarrhal or dry, spasmodic P IV (i) .5 sed.

catarrhal, aggravated by cold air P III (i) .6 sed.

dry, hacking, P IV (i) .16 bis ton.

nervous with dyspnoea P IV (i) .6 ton.

nervous with feeling of tickle in throat P IV (i) .21 & .22 sed

spasmodic P III (i) .11 sed.

spasmodic with dyspnoea P III (i) .10 ton.

whooping

IX.1 (AL IX) sed.

XI.40 (PS-XII) sed.

III.22 (VR VI) sed.

III.13 (VR IX) sed.

CRAMP

abdominal pains P IV (i) .4 sed.

abdominal pains and inflated stomach P IV (i) .9 sed.

of organs, smooth, and striated muscles

VIII.2 (SD) sed. & VIII.3 (RG) sed.

writer's

II.4 (RG) sed.

III.15 (VR I) sed.

CROUP

IX.1 (AL IX) sed.

P IV (i) .20 sed.

CYANOSIS

VIII.3 (RG) sed.

CYSTITIS

III.23 (VR IV) sed.

.27 (VR II) sed.

.28 (VR III) sed.

.64 (RG) sed.

.65 (SD) sed.

IV.4 (PS-III) sed.

P IV (i) .7 (AL VI) sed.

of long standing P IV (i) .4 (AL II) sed.

DEAFNESS
>to human voice,
>after infectious diseases,
>with dental caries,
>incessant noises with vertigo VI.10 (SD) sed.
>All cases of deafness use the following points,
>*with noises*: VI.23 sed. VII.2 sed. VII.3 sed. VI.17 sed.
>P III (i) .19 ton.
>*without noises*: as above, but reverse polarity.

DELIRIUM
>X.4 (RG) sed.
>IX.5 (SD) sed.
>P III (i) .11 sed.
>erotic P IV (i) .7 sed.
>tremens P III (i) .11 sed.

·DEMONIAC POSSESSION IX.5 (SD) sed.

DEPRESSION
>II.3 (TN) ton.
>nervous P III (i) .10 ton.
>(see also psychism points, Chinese System of Healing)

DESPAIR
>P III (i) .19 sed.

DIABETES
>VIII.2 (SD) sed.
>IV.3 (RG) ton.
>VI.4 (RG) ton.
>P III (i) .3 bis sed.
>insipid III.23 (VR IV) ton.
>sugar XI.40 (PS-XII) sed.
>pains in kidneys, local point P III (i).3 bis sed.

DIARRHOEA
>III.21 (VR XI) ton.
>VI.4 (RG) sed.
>VII.43 (TN) ton.
>VIII.2 (SD) sed.
>.3 (RG) sed.
>.14 (AL VIII) sed.
>acute P IV (i) .14 (AL I) sed.
>choleriform X.4 (RG) sed.
>green III.22 (VR VI) sed.
>
>X.2 & .3 (SD) sed.
>XII.15 (AL XII) sed.
>XII.2 (TN) ton.
>P V (i) .6 ton.
>.4 sed.
>.5 sed.

DIGESTION, impaired.   See DYSPEPSIA.

DIGESTION sluggish

     XI.41 (TN) ton.

DIPHTHERIA

     P IV (i) .18 sed.

DISEQUILIBRIUM, physical P III (i) .19 ton.

DISTENSION of tissue by air or gas.   see EMPHYSEMA

DISTRAUGHT

     P III (i) .10bis ton.

DYSENTERY

I.5 (PS-II) sed.	XI.42 (RG) sed.
III.25 (VR X) sed.	XII.2 (TN) ton.
III.27 (VR II) sed.	or .3 (RG) sed.
III.65 (SD) sed.	P IV (i) .3 (AL III) sed.
IV.3 (RG) ton.	P IV (i) .7 (AL VI) sed.
VI.4 (RG) sed.	
VIII.3 (RG) ton.	
VIII.9 (TN) ton.	
acute P IV (i) .14 (AL I) sed.	

DYSMENORRHOEA

     III.15 (VR I) ton.

     III.67 (TN) ton.

     VI.3 (TN) ton.

     VI.4 (RG) ton.

     P IV (i) .3 (AL III) sed.

     P IV (i) .12 (AL VI & XI) sed.

DYSPEPSIA

     IV.1 (SD) sed.

     VIII.9 (TN) ton *or* VIII.14 (AL VIII) sed.

     XI.41 (TN) ton *or* XI.45 (SD) sed.

     XII.15 (AL XII) sed.

     P III (i) .5 sed.

     P IV (i) .7 (AL VI) sed.

     P IV (i) .12 (AL VI & XI) sed.

     chronic P IV (i) .14 (AL I) sed.

     eructations (burning, bitter, acid, fetid)

                           P IV (i) .5 (AL VI) sed.

DYSPHAGIA

     IV.7 (TN) ton *or* IV.2 (SD) sed.

DYSPNOEA

      III.13 (VR IX) ton.
      IV.3 (RG) sed.
      VI.5 (PS-V) sed.
      VI.10 (SD) sed.
      VIII.2 (SD) sed.
      IX.7 (PS-X) sed.
      P IV (i) .5 sed.
      acute P IV (i) .14 (AL I) sed.
      painful P IV (i) .12 (AL XI & VI) sed.
      with nervous cough P IV (i) .6 ton.

DYSURIA

      III.27 (VR II) sed.
        .64 (RG) sed.
        .65 (SD) sed.
      VII.25 (AL IV) sed.
      XII.15 (AL XII) sed.

EAR chronic discharge from. see OTORRHOEA

ECLAMPSIA

      II.4 (RG) sed.
      VIII.3 (RG) sed.
      in puerperium
      II.8 (SD) sed.
      IV.2 (SD) sed.

ECZEMA

      X.11 (TN) ton.
      X.4 (RG) ton.
      XI.4 (TN) ton.
      ears, nose, eyes, P III (i) .10 bis ton.

EMOTIVITY (highly sensitive)

      P IV (i) .6 ton.
      P III (i) .19 ton.
      (see also psychism points, Chinese System of Healing)

EMPHYSEMA
P IV (i) .17 sed.
with asthma IX.9 (TN) ton.

ENDOCARDITIS
I.5 (PS-II) sed.
I.7 (SD) sed. *or* I.9 (TN) ton.
V.1 (AL V) sed.
.6 (PS-VI) sed.
.7 (SD & RG) sed *or* V.9 (TN) ton & V.7 (RG) ton.
all cases IV.3 (RG) sed.
rheumatic I.7 (SD) sed.

ENERGY
depletion, exhaustion, P.IV (i) .6 ton.
loss of physical and moral, P III (i) .13 ton.

ENTERITIS
PIV (i) .6 ton. *or* PIV (i) .12 (AL XI & VI) sed.
duodenal, XII.4 (PS-XI) sed.

ENTEROCOLITIS
P IV (i) .4 (AL II) sed.

EPILEPSY
II.3 (TN) sed.
II.4 (RG) sed.
III.14 (VR V) sed.
III.15 (VR I) sed.
VI.10 (SD) sed.
VIII.2 (SD) sed.
VIII.3 (RG) sed.
IX.5 (SD) sed.
XI.40 (PS-XII) sed.
P III (i) .6 sed.
P III (i) .11 sed.
during periods or in children after trauma II.8 (SD) sed.
in ALL cases P IV (i) .15 ton *or* sed.
see APPENDIX "e" zones.

99

EPISTAXIS
II.3 (TN) ton.
III.15 (VR I) ton *or* III.64 (RG) sed.
IX.5 (SD) sed.
will not stop IV.1 (SD) sed.

ERECTIONS
painful at night P IV (i) .2 sed.
see also PRIAPISM

ERETHISMUS
P IV (i) .5 sed.

EROTOMANIA
P IV (i) .7 (AL VI) sed.
IV.11 (AL V) sed.

ERUCTATIONS
P IV (i) .2 sed.   see DYSPEPSIA

ERYSIPELAS
XI.41 (TN) ton.

EXCITABILITY
excessive P IV (i) .5 sed.
of entire nervous system P III (i) .19 sed.

EXHAUSTION
physical and mental, P III (i) .4 ton.
P IV (i) .6 ton.

EXPECTORATION
fetid P IV (i) .5 sed.

EYELIDS, inflammation of. see BLEPHARITIS

EYE, extreme dilation of pupils, see MYDRIASIS

FACE
blue VIII.3 (SD) sed.
blue almost black IV.1 (SD) sed.
pale VIII.2 (SD) sed.
puffiness of, XI.42 (RG) ton
IX.1 sed.
scarlet, feeling of congestion PIII (i) .19 sed.

FAINTING
II.8 (SD) sed.

FATIGUE
general physical and mental P III (i) .3 (AL III) sed.
due to masturbation P III (i) .6 bis ton.

FEET
cold VIII.3 (RG) sed.
icy cold IV.7 (TN) ton.

FEVER
I.7 (SD & RG) sed.
IX.5 (SD) sed.
alternating hot and cold IX.9 (TN) ton.
cold feeling XI.25 (AL X) sed.
cold feeling, intense X.4 (RG) sed.
intermittent IX.9 (TN) ton.
intermittent and feeling intensely cold IX.42 (RG) ton.
malarial IX.7 (PS-X) sed.
malarial with vomiting VIII.3 (TN & RG) ton.
shivering XI.42 (RG) ton.
shivering followed by sweats V.6 (PS-VI) sed.
sweat little or none VII.37 (PS-VIII) sed.
sweat none IV.3 (RG) ton.
sweats and burning hot skin, sensation of burning in chest
      and back IX.7 (PS-X) sed.
thirst, with great X.4 (RG) ton.
tubercular P IV (i) .4 sed.
typhoid X.4 (RG) ton.

FIBROMA
P IV (i) .4 (AL II) ton.

FISSURE
anal P IV (i) .12 (AL XI & VI) sed.

FISTULA
XI.25 (AL X) sed.
XII.5 (SD) sed.

FLATULENCE
>III.22 (VR VI) sed.
>IV.1 (SD) sed.
>VI.24 (AL VII) sed. *or* VII.43 (TN) ton.
>X.2 & .3 (SD sed.
>XI.41 (TN) ton *or* XI.45 (SD) sed.
>XII.15 (AL XII) sed.
>with colic, diarrhoea P IV (i) .3 sed.

FONTANELLES
>retarded closure P IV (i) .6 ton.

FORGETFULNESS
>I.9 (TN) ton.
>IX.7 (PS-X) sed.
>P III (i) .10 bis ton.

FRACTURES
>P III (i) .3 sed.

FRIGIDITY
>sexual P III (i) .3 bis ton.

FURUNCULUS
>IV.2 (SD) sed.
>VII.38 (SD) sed.

FURUNCULOSIS X.11 (TN) ton.
GALL BLADDER, inflammation of
>see ANGIOCHOLECYSTITIS & CHOLECYSTITIS

GASTRALGIA
>III.22 (VR VI) sed.
>IV.1 (SD) sed *or* IV.7 (TN) ton.
>VI.4 (RG) sed.
>VIII.9 (TN) ton.
>X.2 & .3 (SD) sed.
>XI.24 (AL X) sed) *or* (XI.41 (TN) ton.
>XI.45 (SD) sed   ) *or* (XI.42 (RG) ton.
>XII.2 (TN) ton.   *or* (XII.4 (PS-XI) sed.
>   (XII.15 (AL XII) sed.
>P III (i) .5 sed.
>P IV (i) .12 (AL XI & VI) sed.

GASTRIC
>   feeling of heaviness P IV (i) .3 sed.
>   troubles VII.24 (AL VII) sed.
>   XII.15 (AL XII) sed.
>   P IV (i) .14 (AL) sed.

GASTRITIS
>   V.7 (SD) sed.
>   P IV (i) .13 sed.
>   acute III.21 (VR XI) ton.
>   chronic III.21 (VR XI) sed.

GINGIVITIS
>   XI.45 (SD) sed.

GLANDS
>   sebaceous, inflammation of IV.2 (SD) sed.
>   swelling in neck, P IV (i) .19 sed.
>   see also ADENITIS

GLAUCOMA
>   P III (i) .10 ton.

GLOTTIS
>   spasms of XI.40 (PS-XII) sed.

GLUCAEMIA
>   P III (i) .3 bis sed.

GLYCOSURIA
>   P III (i) .3 bis sed.

GROWING UP TROUBLES
>   XII.5 (SD) sed.

GUMS
>   inflammation of. see GINGIVITIS
>   painful II.9 (SD) sed.

HAEMATEMESIS
>   III.15 (VR I) ton.
>   P IV (i) .5 sed.

HAEMATURIA
III.23 (VR IV) ton.
III.27 (VR II) ton.
VIII.3 (RG) ton.

HAEMOPHILIA
VI.5 (PS-V) sed.

HAEMOPTYSIS
VI.5 (PS-V) sed.
VIII.14 (AL VIII) sed.
IX.7 (PS-X) sed.
XII.15 (AL XII) sed.
P IV (i) .5 (AL VI) sed.

HAEMORRHAGE
XII.15 (AL XII) sed.
VI.5 (PS-V) sed.
P IV (i) .4 (AL II) ton.
followed by weakness VII.43 (TN) ton.
intestinal P IV (i) .4 (AL II) ton.
XII.3 (RG) ton.
P III (i) .6 sed.
uterine IX.7 (PS-X) sed.

HAEMORRHOIDS
III.65 (SD) sed.
  .25 (VR X) sed.
VI.4 (RG) sed.
VII.38 (SD) sed.
XI.45 (SD) sed   ) *or* (XI.41 (TN) ton.
XI.25 (AL X) sed) *or* (XI.42 (RG) ton.
XII.15 (AL XII) sed.
XII.5 (SD) sed.
XII.3 (RG) sed.
P III (i) .4 ton.
P IV (i) .6 ton *or* P IV (i) .5 sed.

HALLUCINATIONS
P III (i) .11 sed.

104

HANDS

palms hot, no sweat V.9 (TN) ton.
icy cold feeling in hands and feet P III (i) .14 ton.

HAY FEVER see ASTHMA

HEADACHES

I.7 (SD) sed.
I.5 (PS-II) sed.
VI.3 (TN) ton *or* VI.4 (RG) sed.
                  VI.5 (PS-V) sed.
VII.43 (TN) ton.
X.2 & .3 (SD) sed *or* X.4 (RG) ton.
XI.45 (SD) sed.
P IV (i) .6 ton.
coming and going, aggravated by touch and movement
                  PIV (i) .4 sed.

occipital, with heavy head
P III (i) .16 sed.

HEART BEAT

abnormally rapid. see TACHYCARDIA
abnormally slow. see BRADYCARDIA
violent with palpitations P IV (i) .12 sed.

HEART

pains P IV (i) .4 sed.

HEAVINESS

feeling of gastric P IV (i) .3 sed.

HEMIPLEGIA

II.3 (TN) ton.
III.15 (VR I) sed.
X.11 (TN) ton.

HEPATIC deficiency VII.40 (RG) ton.

HEPATITIS

P IV (i) .17 (AL VI) sed.

HICCUPS
>XI.40 (PS-XII) sed.
>intractible III.17 sed.

HOARSENESS
>P IV (i) .16 bis ton.

HUNGER
>voracious VI.4 (RG) sed.
>>P IV (i) .5 sed.
>intense but quickly satiated III.21 ton.
>excessive, see BULIMIA

HYDRONEPHROSIS
>VII.25 (AL IV) sed.

HYPERACIDITY
>digestive system P IV (i) .5 sed.

HYPERTENSION
>arterial I.5 (PS-II) sed.
>>IV.2 (SD) & .3 (RG) sed.
>>V.6 (PS-VI) sed.
>>V.7 (SD) sed.
>>XII.15 (AL XII) sed.
>ocular with mydriasis P III (i) .10 ton.

HYPERTROPHY
>cardiac V.1 (AL V) sed.
>>V.7 (SD & RG) sed.
>tonsils VI.4 (RG) ton.

HYPOCHONDRIA
>VIII.9 (TN) ton.

HYPOSYSTOLE
>I.9 (TN) ton.

HYPOTENSION
>arterial V.9 (TN) ton.
>>I.7 (RG) ton.

HYSTERIA
     XI.40 (PS-XII) sed.
     with spasms P III (i) .13 sed.

ICTERUS
     III.18 (VR VIII) sed.
     III.20 (VR XII) sed.
     IV.3 (RG) sed.
     VII.43 (TN) ton.
     VIII.3 (RG) ton.
     XI.45 (SD) sed.

IMPOTENCE
     III.22 (VR VI) ton.
     VI.4 (RG) ton.
     VIII.9 (TN) ton.
     P III (i) .13 bis ton.
     P IV (i) .6 ton.
     complete P III (i) .3 bis ton.

INCONTINENCE
     urine
     III.25 (VR X) ton.
       .64 (RG) ton.
       .67 (TN) ton.
     IV.2 (SD) or IV.7 (TN) ton.
       .4 (PS-III) sed.
     IX.5 (SD) sed.
     chronic III.22 (VR VI) ton.
     nocturnal P IV (i) .3 (AL III) sed.
     or retention of urine P IV (i) .4 (AL II) sed.

INDIFFERENCE
     P III (i) .19 ton.
     IV.7 (TN) ton.

INDIGESTION
     XI.45 (SD) sed.
     see also DYSPEPSIA

INFLAMMATION

of Aorta I.7 (SD & RG) sed.

V.9 (TN) ton.

of bladder. see CYSTITIS

of a bone. see OSTEITIS

of bronchial tubes. see BRONCHITIS

and burning sensation of bladder, ovaries, urethra, vagina,
vulva P IV (i) .7 sed.

of cornea. see KERATITIS

of ear. see OTITIS

of eyelids. see BLEPHARITIS

of gall bladder and bile ducts.

see CHOLECYSTITIS & ANGIOCHOLECYSTITIS

of glands. see ADENITIS

of gums. see GINGIVITIS

of intestine. see ENTERITIS

of a joint. see ARTHRITIS

of larynx. see LARYNGITIS

of a lymph node V.7 (SD) sed.

VIII.3 (RG) sed.

of mastoid process. see MASTOIDITIS

of mouth. see STOMATITIS

of nasopharynx, chronic X.4 (RG) ton.

of periostium. see PERIOSTITIS

of peritonium. see PERITONITIS

of ovary. see OOPHORITIS

of retina. see RETINITIS

of sebaceous glands IV.2 (SD) sed.

of testicle. see ORCHITIS

of urethra and vagina, acute, burning sensation
P IV (i) .5 sed.

of uterus. see METRITIS

INFLUENZA

IX.7 (PS-X) sed.

I.7 (SD & RG) sed.

INJURY

of peripheral nervous system P III (i) .3 sed.

108

INSOMNIA

PIII (i) .19 sed.
P IV (i) .6 ton *or* P IV (i) .12 sed.
see also psychism points, Chinese System of Healing.

INTOLERANCE
P III (i) .13 bis ton.

INTOXICATIONS
III.13 (VR IX) sed.

IRRITABLE
and ill at ease in company of others P III (i) .12 sed.
excessively P III (i) .13 bis ton.
P IV (i) .5 sed.

ITCHING see PRURITIS

JAUNDICE
XII.15 (AL XII) sed.
see ICTERUS

KERATITIS
VI.3 (TN) ton.
X.4 (RG) sed.

KILL
desire to P III (i) .11 sed.

LARYNGITIS
VI.10 (SD) sed.
IX.1 (AL IX) sed.
chronic III.22 (VR VI) sed.
stridulous XI.40 (PS-XII) sed.

LEUCOCYTHAEMIA, LEUKAEMIA
XII.15 (AL XII) sed.
III.20 (VR XII)sed.

LEUCORRHOEA
XI.25 (AL X) sed.
P IV (i) .4 (AL II) ton.

LIPS

    burning VI.4 sed.

LITHIASIS

    IV.7 (TN) ton *or* IV.11 (AL V) sed.
    VII.25 (AL VII) sed *or* VII.40 (RG) ton.
    VII.38 (SD) sed.
    VIII.9 (TN) ton.
    XII.15 (AL XII) sed.
    III.27 (VR II) sed.
    III.28 (VR III) sed.

LIVER

    all affections of VIII.6 (PS-VII) sed.
    when pain on Right Side at inferior angle of scapula
                            VII.23 (AL VII) sed.
    congestion XI.45 (SD) sed.

LOCHIA

    arrested P IV (i) .3 sed.

LUMBAGO

    III.13 (VR IX) sed.
      .28 (VR III) sed.
      .64 (RG) sed.
      .65 (SD) sed.
    XII.3 (RG) sed.
    P III (i) .5 sed.

LUNGS

    feeling of burning weight in P IV (i) .5 sed.

LYMPH NODE

    inflammation of. see **ADENITIS**

MALARIA see PALUDISM

MANIA

    erotic PIV (i) .7 sed.

MANIACAL STATES

    P III (i) .11 sed.

MANIAS
P III (i) .11 bis sed.

MARSH FEVER see PALUDISM

MASTOIDITIS
VI.3 (TN) ton.
XII.2 (TN) ton.

MASTURBATION
chronic P III (i) .3 bis sed.

MATURING DIFFICULTIES
P IV (i) .6 ton.

MEASLES
german (rubella) X.4 (RG) sed.
grave P III (i) .6 sed.

MELANCHOLY
I.7 (SD) sed.
IV.1 & .2 (SD) sed or IV.3 (RG) ton.
IV.7 (TN) ton.

VI.4 (RG) ton.
VII.40 (RG) ton.
VIII.6 (PS-VII) sed.
XI.41 (TN) ton.
XII.2 (TN) ton.
XII.3 (RG) ton.
P III (i) .12 sed or P III (i) .19 ton.

MEMORY, loss of.   see AMNESIA

MENINGITIS
II.4 (RG) sed.
VIII.3 (RG) sed.
IX.5 (SD) sed.

MENOPAUSE
IV.2 (SD) sed.
for Psychological troubles during menopause,
see Chinese System of Healing.

MENORRHAGIA
VIII.2 (SD) sed.

MENSTRUATION, absent. see AMENORRHOEA

MENTAL DISORDERS
IX.9 (TN) ton.
(see also Chinese System of Healing.)

METRITIS
III.22 (VR VI) sed.
III.28 (VR III) sed.
IV.2 (SD) sed.
VI.3 (TN) ton.
X.4 (RG) ton.
XI.25 (AL X) sed.
P IV (i).4 (AL II) sed. *or* P IV (i) .6 ton.
P IV (i).12 (AL XI & VI) sed.
P IV (i) .2 sed.

METRORRHAGIA
VI.10 (SD) sed.
VIII.3 (RG) ton.
XII.15 (AL XII) sed.
P IV (i) .5 (AL VI) sed.

MICTURITION
painful III.18 (VR VIII) sed.
difficulty in, see DYSURIA

MIGRAINE
III.67 (TN) ton.
VI.3 (TN) ton.
VII.24 (AL VII) sed.
P IV (i) .6 ton.
chronic P IV (i) .14 (AL I) sed.

MOUNTAIN SICKNESS
P III (i) .12 sed.

MOUTH
inflammation of P III (i) .12 sed.
dry, with aversion to drinking P III (i) .11 sed.
and pharynx dry, IX.9 (TN) ton.
dry and great thirst VI.4 (RG) ton.

MUCUS
containing pus, flow of. see BLENNORRHAGIA

MUSCLE ACTION
unco-ordinated, see ATAXY.

MYDRIASIS
P III (i) .10 ton.

MYOCARDITIS
I.7 (SD) sed *or* I.9 (TN) ton.
V.6 (PS-VI) sed.

NAUSEA
P IV (i) .3 sed.
P IV (i) .2 sed.
P IV (i) .5 sed.

NECK
swollen glands of
P IV (i) .19 sed.

NEGLIGENT
P III (i) .10bis. ton.

NEPHRITIS
I.9 (TN) ton.
III.23 (VR IV) sed.
III.27 (VR II)sed.
IV.2 (SD) sed.
IV.3 (RG) sed or ton (*an important point*)
VI.10 (SD) sed.
VII.25 (AL VII) sed.
P IV (i) .4 (AL II) sed.
chronic   see BRIGHT'S DISEASE
atrophic from ascendant infection III.58 (PS-IV) sed.
with haematuria IV.11 (AL IV) sed.

NEPHROPTOSIS
VII.25 (AL VII) sed.

NERVES
> to tonify deeply P III (i) .6 bis ton.

NETTLERASH see URTICARIA

NEURALGIA
> II.7 (PS-I) sed.
> II.8 (SD) sed.
> IV.1 & .2 (SD) sed.
> X.4 (RG) sed.
> XII.2 (TN) ton.
> P III (i) .3 sed.

NEURASTHENIA
> IV.3 (RG) sed.
> VI.3 (TN) & VI.4 ton *or* VI.10 (SD) sed.
> P III (i) .3 sed.

NEURITIS
> XII.2 (TN) ton.

NEUROSIS
> III.65 (SD) sed.

NOSE-BLEED see EPISTAXIS

NUTRITION
> defective, see ATHREPSIA

OBSTRUCTION
> intestinal II.3 (TN) ton.

OCCLUSION
> intestinal X.4 (RG) ton.

ODONTALGIA
> P III (i) .15 sed.
> X.4 (RG) sed.
> XI.42 (RG) sed.
> IV.3 (RG) ton.

OEDEMA
P IV (i) .5 (AL VI) sed.
IV.3 (RG) ton.
XI.42 (RG) ton.
face and neck VII.40 (RG) sed.
lungs III.13 (VR IX) ton or sed.
tendency to I.9 (TN) ton.

OLIGURIA
III.21 (VR XI) sed.

ONANISM
inveterate P III (i) .3 bis sed.

OOPHORITIS III.22 (VR VI) ton.

OPTHALMIA NEONATORUM
X.2 & .3 (SD) sed.

ORCHITIS
III.22 (VR VI) ton.

OSTEITIS
XII.5 (SD) sed.

OSTEOMYELITIS
P IV (i) .6 ton.

OTITIS
VI.3 (TN) ton.
VI.4 (RG) ton.
X.4 (RG) ton.
XII.2 (TN) ton.

OTORRHOEA
chronic P IV (i) .6 ton.

OVER-EXCITEMENT
P III (i) .11 sed.

PAIN
acute, to ease P IV (i) .6 ton.
intermittent nerve, see NEURALGIA
in stomach, see GASTRALGIA

115

PALPITATION (cardiac)

      I.7 (SD) sed.   *or* I.9 (TN) ton.

      IV.1 & .2 (SD) sed.)

      followed by   ) *or* IV.7 (TN) ton.

      IV.3 (RG) sed.   )

      V.1 (AL V) sed.

      V.7 (SD) sed.

      XI.45 (SD) sed.

      XII.15 (AL XII) sed.   *or* XII.3 (RG) ton.

      P IV (i) .12 (AL VI & XI) sed.

PALUDISM

      I.7 (SD) sed.

      III.20 (VR XII) sed.) *or* III.64 (RG) ton.

      III.65 (SD) sed.   )

      V.6 (PS-VI) sed.

      VI.3 (TN) ton.   *or* VI.10 (SD) sed.

      IX.7 (PS-X) sed.   *or* IX.9 (TN) ton.

      X.4 (RG) sed.

      XI.42 (RG) ton.

      XII.3 (RG) sed.

      XII.15 (AL XII) sed.

      acute P IV (i) .14 (AL I) sed.

PARALYSIS

      I.5 (PS-II) ton. *special paresis point*

      II.3 (TN) ton.

      II.4 (RG) ton.   *or* II.4 (RG) sed.

      III.14 (VR V) ton.

      VI.10 (SD) sed.

      VIII.3 (RG) ton.

      X.4 (RG) ton.

      X.11 (TN) ton.

      P III (i) .13 ton.

      of bladder P IV (i) .6 ton.

      and impotence in the aged III.64 (RG) ton.

      infantile II.3 (TN) ton.

      spinal origin II.3 (TN) ton.

PARASITES, intestinal

      XI.25 (AL X) sed. coupled with III.21 (VR XI) sed.

PARESIS
       I.5 (PS-II) and I.7 (RG) ton. coupled with
                                  III.15 (VR I) sed.
       III.14 (VR V) ton or sed.
       II.4 (RG) ton.

PARKINSON'S DISEASE
       III.15 (VR I) ton or sed.

PARONYCHIA
       P IV (i) .9 sed.

PEMPHIGUS
       P III (i) .6 bis ton.

PERICARDITIS
       I.7 (SD) sed.   *or* I.9 (TN) ton.
       IV.11 (AL V) sed.
       V.6 (PS-VI) sed.
       V.7 (SD) sed.   *or* V.9 (TN) ton.

PERIODS
       all disturbances of XII.15 (AL XII) sed.
       irregular X.11 (TN) ton.
       premature   P IV (i) .3 sed.
       too long   P IV (i) .3 sed.
       copious   P IV (i) .3 sed.
       late and profuse VIII.6 (see "Bloodmaster" in
                            Chinese System of Healing)

PERIOSTITIS
       XII.5 (SD) sed.
       XI.42 (RG) ton.

PERITONITIS
       II.8 (SD) sed.
       VIII.2 (SD) sed.
       X.4 (RG) ton.
       XI.42 (RG) ton.
       chronic P IV (i) .6 ton.

PHTHISIS. see TUBERCULOSIS, pulmonary

PILES, see HAEMORROIDS
>chronic P IV (i) .6 ton.

PLEURESY
>I.9 (TN) ton.
>IV.2 (SD) sed. and IV.3 (RG) sed.
>VII.43 (TN) ton.
>VIII.2 (SD) sed.
>IX.5 (SD) sed.
>X.2 and .3 (SD) sed.

PNEUMONIA
>III.13 (VR IX) sed.
>IV.2 (SD) and IV.3 (RG) sed.
>VI.10 (SD) sed.
>VI.5 (PS-V) sed.
>IX.5 (SD) sed.
>IX.7 (PS-X) sed.
>IX.9 (RG) sed.

POLYURIA
>III.21 (VR XI) sed.

POSSESSION
>"demoniac" P III (i) .6 sed.

POTTS DISEASE
>III.13 (VR IX) ton.
>P IV (i) .6 ton.

PREGNANCY
>XII.4 (PS-XI) sed.
>discomfort during, acute P IV (i) .14 (AL I) sed.

PRIAPISM
>IV.11 (AL V) sed.
>P III (i) .3 bis sed.
>V.6 (PS-VI) sed.
>P IV (i) .2 sed.
>P IV (i) .7 sed.
>painful, nocturnal P IV (i) .2 sed.

PROLAPSE
 bladder IV.7 (TN) ton.
 rectum XI.25 (AL X) sed.
   XII.4 (PS-XI) sed.
   P III (i) .4 ton.
 uterus XII.4 (PS-XI) sed.

PROSTRATE
 hypertrophy III.28 (VRIII) sed.

PROSTATITIS
 III.18 (VR VIII) sed.
 III.25 (VR X) sed.
 PIV (i) .4 (AL II) sed.

PROSTRATION
 nervous, complete P III (i) .13 ton.

PRURIGO
 III.13 (VR IX) sed.

PRURITIS
 IV.2 (SD) sed.
 P IV (i) .3 (AL III) sed.
 vaginal P IV (i) .7 sed.
 intense P IV (i) .3 (AL III) sed.
 urethra, vulva, P IV (i) .3 and .7 sed.

PSYCHO-NEUROSIS
 XI.40 (PS-XII) sed.

PUSTULES
 P III (i) .6 bis ton.

PYELONEPHRITIS
 III.23 (VR IV) ton.
 VII.25 (AL IV) sed.

PYORRHPEA
 P IV (i) .12 (AL VI and XI) sed.

REFLEXES
 exaggerated P III (i) .13 ter ton.

RESTLESSNESS
P III (i) .19 ton.

RETINITIS
VIII.3 (RG) ton.
VI.10 (SD) sed.

RHEUMATISM
II.7 (PS-I) sed.
IV.1 (SD) sed. followed by IV.2 (SD) sed.
V.6 (PS-VI) sed.
V.1 (AL V) sed.
V.7 (SD and RG) sed.
VIII.2 (SD) sed. *or* VIII.9 (TN) ton.
X.4 (RG) sed.
XI.45 (SD) sed.
P IV (i) .3 (AL III) sed.
deformans II.7 (PS-I) ton.

RHINITIS see CORYZA

RICKETS
XII.5 (SD) sed.
P IV (i) .6 ton.

RUBELLA (epidemic roseola)
X.4 (RG) sed.

RUMBLING
intestinal III.21 ton.

St. VITUS'S DANCE see CHOREA

SADNESS
IV.7 (TN) ton. see also Chinese System of Healing.

SALIVA
copious flow in spite of dry feel in mouth IV.7 (TN) ton.

SATYRIASIS
P III (i) .13 sed.

SCROPHULA
P IV (i) .19 sed.

SEA SICKNESS
P IV (i) .14 sed.

SEBACEOUS GLANDS
inflammation of, IV.2 (SD) sed.

SCIATICA
III.65 (SD) sed.
III.28 (VR III) sed.
VII.40 (RG) sed.
XII.2 (TN) ton.

SCOLIOSIS
III.64 (RG) ton.

SEMANTIC DISTURBANCES
II.3 (TN) ton.

SENILITY
precocious P III (i) .4 ton.

SIALORRHOEA
but tongue and mouth feel dry IV.7 (TN) ton.

SINUSITIS
X.4 (RG) ton.

SKIN
bluish discolouration. see CYANOSIS
dry, hot P IV (i) .13 sed *or* .4 ton.
"skin diseases point" III.54 ton. in centre of the popliteal
space.

SLEEPLESSNESS see INSOMNIA

SOMNAMBULISM
XII.5 (SD) sed.

SPASMS
internal VIII.2 (SD) sed.
oesophagal P III (i) .11 sed.
stomach XI.40 (PS-XII) sed.

SPEAK
inability to, II.3 (TN) ton.
spasmodic inability, see SYSPASIA

121

SPEECH
>extravagant P III (i) .11 sed.
>inability to comprehend II.3 (TN) ton.

SPERMATORRHOEA
>XII.15 (AL XII) sed.
>III.67 (TN) ton.
>nocturnal P IV (i) .6 ton.

SPINE MARROW
>maladies of IV.7 (TN) ton.

SPLEEN
>all affections of XII.15 (AL XII) sed.

STERILITY
>male III.23 (VR) IV ton.
>IV.11 (AL V) ton. *or* IV.1 (SD) sed.
>VI.5 (PS-V) sed.
>VIII.9 (TN) ton.
>P III (i) .3 bis ton.
>P IV (i) .3 (AL III) sed. (male and female)
>>*or* P IV (i) .4 (AL II) ton.

STOMACH
>air or gas in.   see AEROGASTRIA
>inflammation of gastric mucous membrane.
>>see GASTRITIS
>inflated P IV (i) .6 ton.
>pains. see GASTRALGIA

STOMATITIS
>III.22 (VR VI) sed.
>XI.42 (RG) sed.

STOOLS
>discoloured VIII.6 (PS-VII) sed.
>discoloured with golden yellow urine VII.23 (AL VII) sed.
>enteriform, covered with mucous P IV (i) .4 sed.
>undigested matter in, fetid IX.1 sed.

STUPOR
P III (i) .13 bis ton.

SUFFOCATION
feeling of. see ANGINA

SUICIDE
desires and attempts to commit P III (i) .15 sed.

SUPPURATIONS
osseous P IV (i) .9 sed. *or* P IV (i) .6 ton.
tendency to, general VI.3 (TN) ton.

SWALLOWING
difficulty in. see DYSPHAGIA

SWEATS
P III (i) .19 sed.
abundant IV.3 (RG) sed.
little or none VII.37 (PS-VIII) sed.
night V.6 (PS-VI) sed.

SWELLING see ODEMA

SYCOSIS
III.58 (PS-IV) sed.

SYNCOPE
P IV (i) .3 sed.

SYNOVITIS
VIII.2 (SD) sed. and IV.2 (SD) sed.

SYSPASIA
II.3 (TN) ton.

TABES, TABES DORSALIS, see ATAXY

TACHYCARDIA
I.7 (SD) sed.
I.5 (PS-II) sed.
V.7 (SD) sed.

TASTE
bitter in mouth
P IV (i) .2 and .3 sed.
with nausea and vertigo P IV (i) .3 sed.

TEETH
decayed XI.45 (SD) sed.

TESTICLES
swollen and painful.   VIII.6 sed.

TETANUS
II.3 (RG) sed.
III.64 (RG) sed.

THIRST
ardent VI.5 (PS-V) sed.
continuous I.9 (TN) ton.
dry throat X.6 (PS-IX) sed.
intense X.4 (RG) ton.
lively XII.4 (PS-XI) sed.

THOUGHTS
co-ordination of, difficult P III (i) .19 ton.

THROAT
irritations P IV (i) .21 and .22 sed.
dry with thirst X.6 (PS-IX) sed.

TICS
facial IX.5 (SD) sed.

TIMIDITY
P IV (i) .6 ton.

TONE
chronic lack of II.4 (RG) ton.

TONSILITIS
V.7 (SD) sed.
VI.10 (SD) sed.
VII.38 (SD) sed.
X.4 (RG) sed. *or* ton.

TONSILS
   swollen and ulcerated I.7 (SD) sed.

TOOTHACHE see ODONTALGIA

TORTICOLIS
   P III (i) .14 ton. *or* sed.
   III.64 (RG) ton.

TONGUE
   painful and swollen I.9 (TN) ton.
   pale, feels stiff X.4 (RG) sed.
   puffy IX.7 (PS-X) sed.

TRACHOMA
   II.4 (RG) ton.

TRAUMA
   serious in sacro-coccygeal region P III (i) .3 sed.

TRAVEL SICKNESS
   P IV (i) .14 sed.

TREMBLING
   III.15 (VR I) sed.
   IX.5 (SD) sed.

TUBERCULOSIS
   VI.5 (PS-V) sed.
   IX.1 (AL IX) sed.
   VIII.2 (SD) sed.
   IX.7 (PS-X) sed.
   pulmonary IV.1 & .2 (SD) and .3 (RG) sed. (at onset)
   III.13 (VR IX) ton. & III.23 (VR IV) ton.
   IX.9 (TN) ton.
   XII.15 (AL XII) sed.
   vesical IV.4 (PS-III) sed.

TUMOURS
   P IV (i) .4 (AL II) sed.
   P IV (i) .12 (AL VI & XII) sed.

TYPHOID FEVER
III.23 (VR IV) sed.
X.2 & .3 (SD) sed. *or* X.4 (RG) ton.

ULCERS
stomach I.5 (PS-II) sed.
III.22 (VR VI) sed.
III.23 (VR IV) sed.
VI.10 (SD) sed.
XI.45 (SD) & .42 (RG) sed. *or* XI.41 (TN) & .42 (RG) ton.
P III (i) .5 sed.
P IV (i) .5 sed.
varicose XII.5 (SD) sed.

URETHRITIS
P IV (i) .4 sed.
chronic P IV (i) .4 sed.

URICAEMIA
IV.1 (SD) sed.
VIII.9 (TN) ton.

URINE
diminution of secretion, see OLIGURIA
excessive amount passed, see Polyuria
absence of secretion VIII.9 (TN) ton.
retention of P IV (i) .2 sed.

UTERUS
chronic complaints P IV (i) .4 ton.

VAGINA
excoriating burning pains P IV (i) .3 sed.
intense pruritis P IV (i) .3 sed.

VALVULAR
affections, acute I.7 (SD) sed.

VALUES
lost sense of, true and false, P III (i) .12 sed.

VARICOSE
veins, painful XII.5 (SD) sed.
ulcers XII.5 (SD) sed.
veins and haemorroids VII.38 (SD) sed.

VERTIGO

I.5 (PS-II) sed.
III.15 (VR I) sed.
VI.3 (TN) ton. *or* VI.10 (S10) sed.
X.2 & .3 (SD) sed.
XII.15 (AL XII) sed.
P III (i) .19 ton.
P IV (i) .3 sed.

VIGOUR

lack of mental and bodily. see NEURASTHENIA

VOMITING

I.5 (PS-II) sed. *or* II.7 (PS-I) sed.
VI.10 (SD) sed., VI.5 (PS-V) sed.
X.4 (RG) sed.
XI.42 (RG) ton.
XII.2 (TN) ton.
P IV (i) .2 sed., .5 sed.
acute P IV (i) .14 (AL I) sed.
convulsions III.21 (VR XI) sed.
during pregnancy P IV (i) .14 (AL I) sed.
blood. see HAEMATEMESIS
feeling of imminent. see NAUSEA

WEAKNESS

mental P III (i) .10 bis ton.
physical and mental .10 bis ton.
progressive emaciation P IV (i) .6 ton.
profound physical and mental P IV (i) .4 ton.

WHITLOW

P IV (i) .9 sed.

WHOOPING COUGH. see COUGH, whooping

WORMS

intestinal III.67 (TN) ton.

YAWNING

always, and sleepy P III (i) .13 ter ton.

127

HOMOEOPATHIC REMEDIES

CORRESPONDING TO THE CHINESE POINTS

———————

The homoeopathic correspondencies listed, in alphabetical order, are those which have been discovered by Dr. Roger de la Fuÿe and clinically ascertained by him. Some of these remedies had already been discovered by Dr. Weihe: where Dr. de la Fuÿe has clinically confirmed these points he acknowledges it in his text. We have indicated throughout our text the authority for the correspondencies, putting in brackets either (de la Fuÿe) or (Weihe). In this alphabetical list we did not feel it necessary to do this.

Against each remedy, after the potency has been given, we give the meridian number and point, followed, in brackets, the character of the point e.g.: ABROTANUM 3—6, III.21 (VR); HYDRASTIS 6, X.4 (TN); etc. The diagram showing the anatomical position and description of the position may then easily be looked up on the appropriate pages.

Some practitioners, instead of using the repertory, may prefer to decide first what homoeopathic remedies are suitable in the circumstances and then look up the acupuncture point correspondencies. Treatment may then be given by massage, moxa, needles, or remedy in potency, or together.

ABROTANUM	3— 6,	III.21 (VR XI).
ACONITUM	1— 3,	V.9 (TN).
	6— 30,	I.7 (SD & RG).
AETHUSA	3— 6,	III.21 (VR XI).
AGARICUS	6— 30,	III.14 (VR V).
	6— 30,	IX.5 (SD).
ALOE	6— 30,	III.25 (VR X).
	6— 30,	XII.3 (RG).
ALUMINA	6— 30,	II.4 (RG).
	30,	X.II (TN).
AMMON. CARB	3— 6,	IX.9 (TN & RG).
ANTIMON. TAR	6,	X.6 (PS—IX).
	6— 30,	III.13 (VR IX).
ARGENTUM MET	6,	P IV (i) .16 bis.
ARGENTUM NITRICUM	6,	X.2 & .3 (SD).
	6— 30,	III.22 (VR VI).
	6— 12,	P III (i) .5.
ARSEN. ALB.	6— 12,	IV.3 (RG).
	6— 12,	XI.42 (RG).
	6— 30,	XII.2 (TN).
AURUM MET.	30—200,	I.7 (SD & RG).
BERBERIS	3x— 12,	VII.25 (AL IV).
	3— 6,	VII.38 (SD).
	6,	III.19 (VR VII).
	6— 30,	XI.25 (AL X). right side.
BROMIUM	3— 6,	P IV (i) .20
BRYONIA	3— 6,	VIII.2 (SD).
BUFO	30—200,	P III (i) .6 bis.
CACTUS	6,	V.7 (SD & RG).
	6,	V.1 (AL V).
CALCAREA CARB	30—200,	V.6 (PS-VI).
IODATA	6,	P IV (i) .19.
CANTHARIS	6,	III.27 (VR II).
		III.65 (SD).
	6— 30,	IV.11 (AL V).
	6—200,	P IV (i) .7.

129

CARB. SULF	30,	P III (i) .13 bis.
CARBO VEG.	6— 30,	IX.9 (TN & RG).
CEANOTHUS	6— 30,	III.20 (VR XII).
		XII.15 (AL XII) left side.
CHELIDONIUM	3x— 6,	VIII.6 (PS-VII).
	3x— 30,	VII.23 (AL VII).
CHINA	6,	XII.3 (RG).
		VII.43 (TN).
	6— 30,	XII.15 (AL XII) left side.
COCA	6,	P III (i) .12.
COLOCYNTHIS	6,	VII.40 (RG).
CORALLIUM RUBRUM		
	30—200	P III (i) .6.
CRATOEGUS	TM— 3x,	I.7 (SD & RG).
CUPRUM MET.	6— 30,	VIII.3 (RG).
		P IV (i) .13.
	30—200,	II.4 (RG).
CUPRUM ARSEN.	3 —6,	P III (i) .15.
DIGITALIS	6,	I.9 (TN).
EQUISETUM	1x— 6,	IV.4 (PS-III).
FABIANA IMBRICATA		
	TM— 6,	III.18 (VR VIII).
FERRUM IODATUM	3x,	P IV (i) .2.
FERRUM PHOS.	6— 12,	IX.5 (SD).
FLUORICUM ACIDUM		
	12— 30,	XII.5 (SD).
GELSEMIUM	6,	III.15 (VR I). left side.
GINSENG	TM,	V.7 (SD & RG).
	TM— 3x,	P III (i) .3 bis.
	I— 3,	V.9 (TN).
GRAPHITES	3x— 6x,	XI.41 (TN).
HEPAR SULF.	6,	IX.1 (AL IX).
HYDRASTIS	6,	X.4 (RG).
	6— 30,	P IV (i) .4.
HYDROPHOBINUM	30—200,	P III (i) .11.
HYPERICUM	3x— 6,	P III (i) .3.
IODIUM	6, 30, 200,	P IV (i) .11 bis.
IPECA	6— 12,	P IV (i) .14.

KALI CARB.	3x— 12,	III.67 (TN).
	6,	III.15 (VR I) right side.
	6— 30,	VII.24 (AL VII).
LATHYRUS SATIVUS	30,	P III (i) .13 bis.
LYCOPODIUM	6— 12,	IV.1 (SD).
		VII.40 (RG).
	12— 30,	VIII.9 (TN).
MEDORRHINUM	6 —M,	III.58 (PS-V).
MENYANTHES	6— 30,	P III (i) .14.
MERCURIUS IOD RUB	6,	P IV (i) .18.
MERCURIUS SOLUBILIS		
	6— 30,	IV.7 (TN).
MEZERUM	30,	P IV (i) .11.
MOSCHUS	3— 6,	XI.40 (PS-XII).
MUREX	30,	P III (i) .3 bis.
		V.7 (SD & RG).
	200,	V.7 (SD & RG).
MYRICA	3— 12,	VII.37 (PS-VIII).
NAJA	6,	V.7 (SD & RG).
NITRICUM ACIDUM	6,	XI.42 (RG).
NUX MOSCHATA	30,	VIII.14 (AL VIII).
NUX VOMICA	6— 12,	XI.45 (SD).
	6— 30,	XII.15 (AL XII) right side.
		III.65 (SD).
OENANTHE CROCATA		
	6— 30,	II.8 (SD).
OPIUM	30— M,	X.4 (RG).
ORIGANUM	6,	P III (i) .3 bis.
		V.7 (SD & RG).
	30,	V.7 (SD & RG).
OSMIUM	30—200,	P III (i) .10.
PARIS QUADRIFOLIA	30,	P III (i) .11 bis.
PHOSPHORIC ACID	3, 6, 30,	P IV (i) .15.
PHOSPHORUS	6,	VI.5 (PS-V).
		IX.7 (PS-X).
	6—30,	I.5 (PS-II).
		IV.3 (RG).
		VI.10 (SD).
		P III (i) .16.

		P IV (i) .5.
	200—M,	VIII.3 (RG).
PICRICUM ACIDUM	6— 30,	P III (i) .13.
PLUMBUM	30—200,	II.3 (TN).
PODOPHYLLUM	6—12,	XII.4 (PS-XI).
PSORINUM	30— M,	VI.4 (RG).
RAPHANUS SATIVUS	6,	P IV (i) .17.
RHUS RADICANS	6,	P III (i) .16.
RHUS TOX	3— 12,	P IV (i) .3.
RUMEX CRISPUS	3— 6,	P IV (i) .21 & .22.
SANGUINARIA	6,	IX.9 (TN & RG).
SELENIUM	30— M,	P III (i) .4.
SEPIA	6— 12,	XII.4 (PS-XI).
	6— 30,	IV.7 (TN).
	30,	XI.25 (AL X) left side.
SILICEA	30—200	P IV (i) .9.
		XII.5 (SD).
	30— M,	VI.3 (TN).
	200— M,	P IV (i) .6.
SPIGELIA	3— 6,	V.7 (SD & RG).
STAPHYSAGRIA	6— 30,	V.7 (SD & RG).
	200,	P III (i) .3 bis.
	200—DM,	V.7 (SD & RG).
STRAMONIUM	30—200,	P III (i) .11.
SULPHUR	30—200,	IV.2 (SD).
	30— M,	VI.4 (RG).
TABACUM	12— 30,	P IV (i) .14.
TELLURIUM	200— M,	P III (i) .10 bis.
TEREBENTHINA	6— 12,	III.23 (VR IV).
THERIDION	30—200,	P III (i) .19.
THUYA	6, 30, 200,	P IV (i) .12.
URANIUM NITRICUM		
	6—200,	P III (i) .3 bis.
VERATRUM ALBUM	3— 6,	P IV (i) .14 bis.
	6,	X.4 (RG).
	6— 30,	II.7 (PS I).
ZINCUM MET.	30—200,	P III (i) .19.

The French text is quoted from Principe Unique de la Philosophie et de la Science d'Extrême-Orient, par Nyoiti Sakurazawa, 1958, by kind permission of the publishers, Librairie Philosophique J. Vrin, 6, Place de la Sorbonne, Paris Ve. pages 35 and 36.

LA LOI UNIQUE

The Unique Law

Loi Unique: "L'univers, c'est l'oscillation des deux activitiés In et Yo, et ses vicissitudes":

ONE LAW: The universe represents the oscillation of the two activities, Yin and Yang, and their vicissitudes.

1. Ce qui produit et compose l'univers est Taikyoku (L'univers-éther, ou la nature intime, Çûnyatâ en sanscrit: Kû en japonais).

    That which produces and composes the universe is Taikyoku (universe-ether, or inner nature, Çûnyatâ in Sanscrit: Kû in Japanese).

2. Taikyoku se polarise: un pôle se charge d'activité Yo, l'autre d'activité In.

    Taikyoku polarises: one pole becomes charged with Yang activity, the other with Yin activity.

3. L'activité Yo (constrictrice, d'ou chaleur, pesanteur centripète) et l'activité In (dilatatrice, d'où le froid, force d'ascension) sont opposées.

    Activity Yang (constrictive, from whence heat, weight centripetal) and activity Yin (dilating, from whence cold, force of ascension) are opposites.

4. Les êtres et les phénomènes qui se produisent dans l'univers sont des agrégats multiples et complexes de substance Taikyoku chargée des deux activités In et Yo en toutes proportions. (Notre univers lui-même n'est autre chose qu'une partie infime de cette manifestation de Taikyoku.)

Beings and phenomena occurring in the universe are multiple and complex aggregates of Taikyoku substance charged with Yin and Yang activities in all proportions. (Our universe itself is none other than a lowest ranking level of this Taikyoku manifestation.)

5. Les êtres et les phénomènes sont des équilibres dynamiques divers; rien n'est stable ni fini dans l'univers, tout est en mouvement incessant, parce que la polarisation, la source des êtres, est sans commencement ni fin.

Beings and phenomena are diverse dynamic equilibra; nothing in the universe is stable or finished, all is in unceasng motion, because polarisation, the source of beings, is without beginning and without end.

6. L'activité In et l'activité Yo s'attirent l'une l'autre.

Yin activity and Yang activity attract one another.

7. Rien n'est In absolue, ni Yo absolu. In et Yo ne se caractérisent que relativement; tout est agrégat de In et Yo.

Nothing is wholly Yin nor wholly Yang. Yin and Yang are characterised only relatively: all is Yin and Yang aggregate.

8. Rien n'est neutre. La polarisation est incessante et universelle.

Nothing is neutral. Polarisation is ceaseless and everywhere.

9. La force d'attraction entre deux êtres est fonction de la différence entre leurs charges d'activês opposees.

The force of attraction between two beings is a function of the difference between their charges of opposite activities.

136

10. Les activités de même nom se repoussent. La répulsion entre deux êtres de même activité est d'autant plus grande qu'ils sont plus proches.

Like activities repel one another. The repulsion between two beings of the same activity is the greater the closer they are.

11. In produit Yo; Yo produit In.

Yin produces Yang; Yang produces Yin.

12. Tous les êtres se chargent d'activité: Yo à l'intérieur, et In à l'extérieur.

All beings are charged: Yang interiorly, Yin exteriorly.

APPENDIX   B

Sympatheticotonia and the "e" zones

Sympatheticotonia is the name given by Dr. Wilhelm Reich to a long continued general state of anxious muscular contraction: the basic characteristic being a chronic inspiratory attitude of the thorax limiting full expiration.*

Energy producton is directly proportionate to efficient respiration: for the function of breathing is (a) to introduce into the organism the oxygen required for the combustion of digested food, producing vegetative energy, and, (b) the elimination of the waste product of combustion, carbon-dioxide. Inhibited breathing results in a reduced intake of oxygen, and retention of excess CO_2 in the system. Among other areas of tension occuring in sympatheticotonia should be mentioned these: head and neck muscles, mouth chin and throat muscles.

According to Reich, chronic sympatheticotonia leads to general disturbances of vegetative equilibrium, leading to disorders such as: Violent headaches (frontal, occipital, and behind the eyes), cardiovascular hypertension, tachycardia, hyperthyroidism, rheumatism, lumbago, chronic constipation (resulting from chronic spasm of anal sphincter), vaginismus, chorea, epilepsy, etc.

Reich points out that there are certain areas of the skin surface, characterized by an extremely variable intensity of sensation and capacity of excitation, showing fundamentally different behaviour from the rest of the skin surface. Experiments were carried out by Reich and a team of other scientific researchers at the Psychological Institute of the University of Oslo, 1935 and 1936. The results were

* W. Reich, Discovery of Orgone, chapter VIII on the orgasm reflex and the technique of character-analytic vegetotherapy, pp234 et seqq.

published in a monograph: Experimentille Ergebnisse über die elektrische Funktion von Sexualität und Angst. Sexpol Verlag 1937. These experiments involved a stimulation *closely allied to a very delicate Chinese sedative massage.* The cutaneous areas concerned are called "erogenous" zones, namely: lips, anus, nipples, penis, mucous membrane of the vagina, earlobe, tongue, palms of the hands, and forehead. We refer to these as the "e" zones.

The "e" zones for *present* consideration are the following: lips, earlobe, palms, forehead.

There are Chinese acupuncture points on these "e" zones (organ meridians and vessel meridians). Twelve of these points are bilateral and three median. To these we have added one median point. *Not one of these points is ever mentioned by Dr. de la Fuÿe in his Traité d'Acupuncture.*

In Akupunktur als Neuraltherapie Dr. Stiefvater indicates as NOT USED the following: I.8, IX.10, P III (i) .26. He names, but gives no symptoms nor treatment indication for the following: II.19, VII.9, .10, & .11. For the remaining points he gives symptoms treated at these points; III.3, .4, .5, V.8, VII.4, XI.1, P.III (i) .22 and .23.

P IV (i).25 is not included in the traditional meridians. This point we have named TCHRENG-TSIANG bis, and placed the anatomical position at the centre of the lower lip at the place where, when the lips are closed, the point P III (i) .26 is in contact.

The six bilateral points and the one median point on the forehead for which Stiefvater gives therapeutic indications are the following:

III.3   MEI-TCHRONG

anatomical position: bilateral, about 7 cm. above the supra-orbital foramen, on the junction of the epicranial aponeurosis and the frontal portion of the occipito-frontalis muscle.

Treatment: needle 2mm.

Indications and symptoms: Epilepsy, Headache, Common Cold.

III.4 TSIOU-TCHRAE
anatomical position: bilateral, 2 cm horizontally lateral to .3.

Treatment: needle 2 mm.

Indications and symptoms: Nose-bleed, heart complaints.

III.5 OU-TCHROU
anatomical position: bilateral, 4 cm above .4.

Treatment: needle 2 mm.

Indications and symptoms: Convulsions, tensions in spinal region, pain in region of kidneys.

V.8 LAO-KONG
anatomical position: bilateral, on the palm of the hand, on the lateral border of the flexor tendon of the middle finger (on the crease of the flexed hand).

Treatment: needle 1—2 mm. (NOT DEEPER).

Indications and symptoms: Epilepsy, Disturbed sensitivity of hand, Migraines, nose bleeds, pain in the breasts, great thirst, hypertonicity.

VII.4 RANN-IA
anatomical position: bilateral, on the frontal bone, at the suture of sphenoid and parietal bones (Pterion).

Treatment: needle 1—3 mm.

Indications and symptoms: Migraine, Epilepsy, Hemiplegia, Eye pains, Blindness, Articular Rheumatism.

XI.1 TREOU-OE
anatomical position: bilateral, on the frontal protruberance.

Treatment: needle 1—3 mm.

Indications and symptoms: Cerebral congestion, Hemiplegia, Violent headaches, facial paralysis, Wind causes flow of tears.

P III (i) .22   TCHROANG-ROE

anatomical position: median, on the frontal bone, 3 cm from the meeting of the saggital suture and frontal bone.

Treatment: needle 2 mm.

Indications and symptoms: Cerebral congestion. Inflammation of the muscles of the nose.

P III (i) .23   CHENN-TING

anatomical position: median, on the frontal bone, halfway between bregma and glabella.

Treatment: needle 2 mm.

Indications and symptoms: Headache, Epilepsy, Running cold.

The similarity of indications and symptoms given by Reich to those according to Acupuncture tradition appears to us to be too close to be passed off as "co-incidence". It does not appear unreasonable to us to suggest that *controlled experiments using acupuncture treatment at the other points on the "e" zones as well* might show the "e" zone points to be suitable for *effective* treatment of sympatheticatonia and resultant disorders.

Tunbridge Wells 1959